MW00962423

Permanent Habit Control

Practitioner's Guide to Using Hypnosis and Other Alternative Health Strategies

To Judy:
My mentor, colleague
& friend... I look
forward to future collaborations
& much fun!
David
March 2016

Brian S. Grodner, PhD, ABPP, FAClinP, is a board-certified, licensed clinical and organizational psychologist and Clinical Assistant Professor at the University of New Mexico College of Medicine. He received his PhD from the University of New Mexico, 1975, and is diplomate in Clinical Psychology, American Board of Professional Psychology. A Fellow of the Academy of Clinical Psychology, he is also the Director of the Enneagram Institute of New Mexico, serves as a certified Enneagram teacher (Riso-Hudson), and is the Director of the Milton Erickson Institute for Clinical Hypnosis and Behavioral Sciences of New Mexico. He has been in private practice for 35 years and is a certified trainer and conductor of hypnosis and counseling to help clients with weight loss and smoking cessation, peak performance (in the area of sports psychology), psychotherapy, energy psychology therapies, EMDR (eye movement desensitization reprocessing), and much more. Furthermore, he is Master Practitioner and Trainer for the Neuro-linguistic program (NLP).

David B. Reid, PsyD, is a licensed clinical psychologist, author, Adjunct Clinical Professor in the Department of Health Sciences at the James Madison University, and Founder and President of In The Zone Consulting, Inc., a business consulting firm in Central Virginia specializing in leadership training, conflict resolution, and promotion of healthy workplace habits. A graduate of Loyola College in Maryland and Wright State University, Dr. Reid completed a postdoctoral fellowship in rehabilitation and neuropsychology at the University of Virginia in 1993. In 2005, Dr. Reid was selected and appointed by Governor Mark Warner of Virginia to serve on the Commonwealth Neurotrauma Initiative (CNI) Trust Fund Advisory Board, a governor-appointed body that administers the funding of ground-breaking medical research and innovative community-based rehabilitation programs in the field of acquired neurotrauma. He was elected chairman of the CNI during his first year and was recently reappointed to this board by Governor Tim Kaine. Dr. Reid has appeared as a guest on radio and television news programs and served as an expert behavioral health consultant to an ABC affiliate in Harrisonburg, Virginia.

Permanent Habit Control

Practitioner's Guide to Using Hypnosis and Other Alternative Health Strategies

Brian S. Grodner, PhD, ABPP, FAClinP
David B. Reid, PsyD

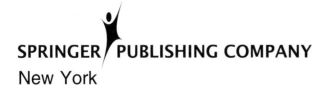

SPRINGER PUBLISHING COMPANY
New York

Copyright © 2010 Springer Publishing Company, LLC

All rights reserved.

No part of this publication may be reproduced, stored in a retrieval system, or transmitted in any form or by any means, electronic, mechanical, photocopying, recording, or otherwise, without the prior permission of Springer Publishing Company, LLC, or authorization through payment of the appropriate fees to the Copyright Clearance Center, Inc., 222 Rosewood Drive, Danvers, MA 01923, 978-750-8400, fax 978-646-8600, info@copyright.com or on the Web at www.copyright.com.

Springer Publishing Company, LLC
11 West 42nd Street
New York, NY 10036
www.springerpub.com

Acquisitions Editor: Philip Laughlin
Production Editor: Pamela Lankas
Cover Design: TG Design
Composition: International Graphic Services

Ebook ISBN: 978-0-8261-0388-8

10 11 12 13 / 5 4 3 2 1

The author and the publisher of this Work have made every effort to use sources believed to be reliable to provide information that is accurate and compatible with the standards generally accepted at the time of publication. Because medical science is continually advancing, our knowledge base continues to expand. Therefore, as new information becomes available, changes in procedures become necessary. We recommend that the reader always consult current research and specific institutional policies before performing any clinical procedure. The author and publisher shall not be liable for any special, consequential, or exemplary damages resulting, in whole or in part, from the readers' use of, or reliance on, the information contained in this book. The publisher has no responsibility for the persistence or accuracy of URLs for external or third-party Internet Web sites referred to in this publication and does not guarantee that any content on such Web sites is, or will remain, accurate or appropriate.

Library of Congress Cataloging-in-Publication Data

Grodner, Brian S.
    Permanent habit control : practitioner's guide to using hypnosis and other alternative health strategies / Brian S. Grodner and David B. Reid.
       p. ; cm.
    Includes bibliographical references and index.
    ISBN 978-0-8261-0387-1 (alk. paper)
    1. Hypnotism—Therapeutic use. 2. Habit breaking. I. Reid, David B. II. Title. [DNLM: 1. Behavior Therapy—methods. 2. Habits. 3. Hypnosis. 4. Personality Assessment. WM 425 G873p 2009]
RC495.G763 2009
615.8'512—dc22
                                        2009050287

Printed in the United States of America by Hamilton Printing.

Contents

Preface

Quitting smoking is easy. I've done it hundreds of times.
—Mark Twain

It has been said that old habits die hard. Every day you can witness the frustration and powerlessness of an individual surrendering to a hard-to-break habit that seems to control her more than she controls it. Whether the persistent behavior involves nail biting, smoking, over-eating, alcohol abuse, drug addiction, or compulsive shopping, the pesky habit claims victory in the end regardless of the resistance or efforts employed to ward it off. And the excuses rendered following defeat are all too familiar and convenient: "I can't help it," "I don't even know I'm doing it," "It's so automatic," "I've tried everything!" and "Nothing works!"

Perhaps you've tried to break an old habit, or maybe committed to a New Year's resolution only to have it transform from personal conviction to fiction within a matter of weeks. According to an informal survey of Pittsburgh residents, five of the top ten 2007 New Year's resolutions involved undoing or breaking some unwanted habit (Powell & Powell, 2007). And no matter how certain or confident a person feels about his intention to change his behavior, odds are most New Year's resolutions will be broken within 14 days! Based on these statistics alone, it's no wonder we believe that old habits die hard.

One of David's clients, Mary, was no different. Her New Year's resolution for the past six years was to quit smoking. One year she made it 10 consecutive days and was on a roll until the day her cat died. After discovering her expired cat, Lola, curled up like a lifeless furry pillow at the foot of her bed, she ran to the kitchen, retrieved her hidden pack of Marlboros and reinitiated a habit of cigarette smoking that seemed unbreakable. That is, until the day she found herself sitting in front of her television set 2 years later as Tom Brokow informed his viewers about the latest study indicating women smokers were more likely to die from breast cancer than their nonsmoking peers. Staring at the lit cigarette dangling between her fingers, she pondered life as a 35-year-old married mother of two young children, and suddenly felt all alone. She had buried her mother 3 days earlier and knew if she didn't kick the habit soon enough, her children would be mourning her loss as well. Her mother had celebrated her 55th birthday 1 week before succumbing to a massive heart attack that took her life. The doctor delivering the tragic news told Mary it was the cigarettes and morbid obesity that killed her. With vivid images of her mother's casket being lowered into a freshly dug grave, Mary pondered that next drag off her cigarette and all it could do to her. Usually, she eagerly anticipated what it would do *for* her: calm frazzled nerves, thwart a looming panic attack, offer momentary, if false, respite. Now she fretted about what it would do *to* her. She snuffed the cigarette into an ashtray, determined it was the last one she would ever smoke. After all, she didn't want to become a permanent nonsmoker in the same way her mother had. But Mary was already 75 pounds overweight, and the notion of packing on more weight (apparently a given when one quits smoking) was enough to restart the habit she'd quit only seconds before. She reconsidered her plan of tossing the remains of her last pack into the trash can. It was like saying "goodbye" to an old friend, just like she had when she buried her mother. Now she *needed* a cigarette. And a cigarette she had.

Like most smokers, Mary tried just about every treatment intervention known to mankind to help her kick the habit. She'd tried all the nicotine replacement options: the patch, the gum, a nasal spray, even an inhaler. One time, she responded to an ad in the Sunday newspaper espousing hypnosis as the way to uproot and resolve the source of her addiction. Having little to lose and a life to live, she paid the nonrefundable registration fee and joined a group of other desperate smokers crammed into a claustrophobic classroom of a local elementary school hoping this would do the trick. She sat perfectly still, catatonic-like, her eyes shut off to external distractions from the outside world, while a certified hypnotist (more on that later) did his thing, offering one hypnotic suggestion after another to her subconscious mind. To the best of her ability, she resisted the urge to resist. Before she knew it, her left hand was rising off her lap and, without conscious intention, levitating in midair. She thought about how ridiculous she and everyone else must have looked with one arm frozen in space, then dismissed the concern, realizing that, if it would actually help her quit smoking, she'd cluck like a chicken if the hypnotist commanded it. Three days later Mary found herself $85 poorer and up to one-and-a-half packs of cigarettes a day.

Sadly, Mary's story isn't unique. In fact, cigarette smoking continues to be identified as the most important preventable cause of death and disease in the United States, with more than one out of every six American deaths resulting from primary or secondary effects of smoking (Centers for Disease Control and Prevention, 2002). According to the National Institutes of Health (2006), of the 44.5 million adult smokers in the United States, 70% want to quit and 40% make a serious quit attempt each year, but in any given year fewer than 5% succeed.

Although the number of smokers in most segments of our population has declined since the late 1990s, recent surveys of middle and high school student smokers have not produced such optimistic findings (Centers for Disease Control and Prevention, 2006). Each day, nearly 4,000 teens smoke their first cigarette, most by age 15, with another 2,000 becoming regular, daily smokers before their eighteenth birthday (Substance Abuse and Mental Health Services Administration, 2006).

Like teen smoking, the prevalence of overweight children and adolescents, and obesity among men in particular, increased significantly from 1999 to 2004 (Ogden et al., 2006). With the alarming increase in morbidly obese people in the world, public health officials have now identified obesity as an epidemic and, sad to say, are commonly referring to our culture as "obesogenic."

Unlike smokers, whose limited options for kicking the habit include quitting cold-turkey, swallowing a pill, or slapping a nicotine replacement patch on their shoulder, overweight and obese individuals do not lack for resources, information, or interventions to assist them with shredding excess poundage. A quick scan of any television program schedule nearly any time of the day reveals a plethora of weight loss/ fitness programs, ranging from infomercials selling appetite suppressants and fat-burning concoctions to home gyms and body buffing contraptions guaranteed to turn any beer-belly gut into a set of rock-solid six-pack abs in record time. But wait, there's more if you order right now! (Just kidding.) A quick jaunt to the local Barnes and Noble or an online surfing session at Amazon.com will offer any interested customer an abundance of best selling reference works on the latest diets and weight loss programs that come and go like the seasons of the year. Unfortunately, the quick-fix options flooding the media and force-fed to the masses have done little to promote a culture of health and fitness. Instead, rather than offering viable solutions for trimming our ever-expansive waistlines, it seems proactive entrepreneurs have taken advantage of a ripe opportunity to sell their wares to a desperate "obesogenic" culture.

Although individual choice and control over one's own destiny, including one's health and well-being, should be respected, maintaining an attitude of lackadaisical bystander apathy to the direct and indirect consequences of smoking and obesity will, over time, pose dire consequences that our society can ill afford. Adverse consequences of smoking and overeating affect all of us and, as surprising as this may seem, extend beyond the smoker or obese individual. This point was driven home after a government study published in the *American Journal of Preventive Medicine* reported that the airline industry spent nearly $275 million to burn 350 million more gallons of fuel in the year 2000 just to carry the additional weight of American passengers (Dannenberg, Burton, & Jackson, 2004). And a recent comprehensive evaluation of 22 independent studies investigating the adverse effects of secondhand smoke in the workplace in the United States, Canada, Europe, China, Japan, and India reported a 50% increased risk of lung cancer for exposed nonsmokers (Stayner et al., 2007). Although smoking is banned in most workplaces in the United States, according to the 2006 Surgeon General's report, nonsmokers working in bars, cafes, and restaurants are chronically exposed to secondhand cigarette smoke throughout their workday and remain at significant risk for cancer and other respiratory illnesses (U.S. Department of Health and Human Services, 2006).

There is also widespread concern among medical experts that the escalating number of morbidly obese children and adults over the next decade will cause health care expenditures in the United States to climb exponentially. These concerns have already become a reality, as medical expenses for morbidly obese adults in the year 2000 were 81% greater than for normal-weight adults, 65% more than for overweight adults, and 47% more than for "merely" obese adults (Arterburn, Maciejewski, & Tsevat, 2005).

It is apparent from these statistics, and from the limited sustained efficacy of current treatment interventions for smoking cessation and weight management, that alternative strategies are necessary to help people like Mary become permanent nonsmokers and permanently slim and fit individuals. In *Permanent Habit Control: Practitioner's Guide to Using Hypnosis and Other Alternative Health Strategies* (henceforth *Permanent Habit Control*), we offer a one-of-a-kind professional resource that provides eclectic and innovative behavioral and naturalistic interventions that can be individually tailored and applied to help your clients become *permanent* nonsmokers and/or *permanently* slim and fit individuals.

Most weight-loss and smoking-cessation programs offer a means to an end (e.g., not smoking, losing 40 pounds) that merely begins a new vicious cycle that simply promotes more of the same (e.g., smoking, weight gain). In general, fad diets, short-lived exercise programs, or a self-adhesive nicotine patch are almost destined to fail, since they rely exclusively on external solutions to an identified "problem" while ignoring the essential skills and resources that reside within all of us that can facilitate and foster change.

Permanent Habit Control is the first book of its kind to employ the Enneagram—a profound psychological and spiritual tool for understanding ourselves and offering pragmatic insight to initiate and promote change in our lives—to help people become permanent nonsmokers and permanently fit and trim. In conjunction with hypnosis and Energy Psychology interventions, we will show you how to utilize the Enneagram to provide essential information concerning your client's personality and behavioral traits that are notoriously overlooked or minimized in most weight loss and smoking cessation programs. This book does not require any prior experience or training in clinical hypnosis, the Enneagram, or exposure to the field of Energy Psychology to be of benefit to you. Rather, we will provide you with all the requisite guidance and information needed to learn and confidently apply all of the strategies and interventions described in this book to help your clients initiate positive and permanent habit change in their lives.

Throughout our book, we draw on case histories from our own clinical work to illustrate the interventions in practical and strategic ways. At the end of each chapter, we invite you to participate in activities designed to enhance and supplement your learning experience. These hands-on, nonthreatening opportunities will help you incorporate new strategies and interventions into your clinical work immediately. From the generation of an individualized treatment plan to the application of personality assessment results obtained from the Riso-Hudson Enneagram Type Indicator (RHETI; Riso & Hudson, 2003), case studies bring life to specific treatment interventions for enhancing habit control.

If it is indeed true that old habits die hard, it might seem that the work to undo them would be tedious, time-consuming, frustrating, and near impossible. As you can likely gather from the title of our book, however, we don't hold this old adage to be fact. Though unwanted habits may be difficult to modify, they don't have to be. We maintain that by understanding the relationship between a habit and its source of reinforcement, and by helping people access and mobilize personal resources that have previously remained unavailable to them or perhaps simply forgotten, habits are not only malleable, but can be replaced by healthier behaviors that enhance the likelihood of permanent habit control.

It is our expectation that, as you follow along in this book, you will have ample opportunities to apply the knowledge and information contained within to help your clients manage what have conventionally been considered difficult-to-treat behaviors. As a "bonus," of sorts, we would also encourage you to select and treat your own personal unwanted habit(s) that you are motivated to change.

USING THIS BOOK

Much work and research in the area of habit control has traditionally focused on external factors by relying predominantly on behavioral techniques, manipulation of the environment, implementation of restrictions, or solicitation of external support. Rather than focus attention and treatment efforts exclusively on external solutions, which are indeed important, we will explore in detail how habit control can be made permanent predominantly by mobilizing and accessing internal resources.

Accomplishing this task depends upon many factors that will be discussed throughout this book. We share specific strategies, processes, metaphors, images, reframing techniques, task assignments, and other innovative techniques for managing unwanted habits, beginning with the initial client contact and continuing through relapse prevention and follow-up reinforcement sessions.

With regard to client assessment, we offer more strategies and techniques than you will probably use for any one client, but this intentional thoroughness will allow you to determine what works best for you and meets each client's specific needs.

Since we focus our attention on weight control and smoking cessation throughout this book, we have interspersed examples addressing both issues. Often, whatever is applied to one habit can be successfully applied to the other. Sometimes, though, specific interventions may be more relevant to smoking cessation than to weight control, and vice versa. For example, nicotine withdrawal is obviously something that is relevant to smoking cessation but not to weight management, whereas a healthy diet and exercise are essential for weight management but will be of little use for smoking cessation.

In essence, to generate permanent habit change, we must shift the ratio of the "no" that comes from hesitation, doubt, and inner conflict impacting our desire and ability for change, to the "yes" that occurs when all aspects of change are strong, aligned, and congruent. We believe people are genuinely interested in changing, but there is a preponderance of problems, including limited motivation, poor initiative, inertia, and disappointment, that challenges desired change. We consequently help our clients systematically shift the ratio from "No, I don't think I can do this" to a YES response set of "I can and I will do this." Rather than spend energy and focused attention on what our client *doesn't want* (e.g., gain more weight, become irritable, fail) we help them gain confidence in their ability to focus energy and attention on what they *do want* (e.g., becoming a permanent nonsmoker).

When conceptualizing and organizing this book, we decided to divide it into three separate but interdependent sections, starting with **Setting the Stage**, which includes a guideline for focused habit assessment to supplement a standard intake interview, an introduction to the Enneagram, and two chapters overviewing the importance of soliciting reasons for change as well as reasons that continue to promote unhealthy and unwanted habits.

In the second section, **Teach Them and Let Them Lead the Way**, we teach you how to teach your clients pragmatic and effective interventions that will help them access and mobilize resources, including those subconsciously relegated to presently inaccessible areas of the mind as well as others that have never been identified or developed. And, as the title of this section implies, we also provide you with no-nonsense psychobabble-free information concerning the consequences of smoking and obesity to share with your clients. Finally, this section provides suggestions for homework assignments that generate and sustain momentum for change, taking the lesson from the clinic to the real world.

In the last section, **May the Force Be With You**, we introduce you to the clinical tools that we have relied on over the years to help our clients make the permanent habit changes they are seeking: Hypnosis, Mindfulness, Energy Psychology, and Emotional Freedom Techniques (EFT). During this section we also bring everything together by utilizing the Enneagram of Personality Types to guide our treatment of two representative clients.

For some people, when it comes to "alternative" or "unconventional" therapeutic interventions like hypnosis or Emotional Freedom Techniques, they need to see it to believe it. We suggest (and yes, it's only a suggestion) that you set aside any of your own "Doubting Thomas" feelings for the moment and consider the possibility that maybe, just maybe, when you *believe* it, then you'll *see* it.

We hope your experience working along with us not only enhances your clinical practice, but your own life as well. If you are so inclined, let us know how you are progressing and drop us a line at David's e-mail address: dreid@drdavidreid.com.

Let's get started.

Acknowledgments

My greatest professional influence has been Dr. Milton Erickson, the great psychiatrist and hypnotherapist with a brilliant mind and warm heart. Dr. Fritz Perls, the founder of Gestalt Therapy, and other Gestalt therapists were the source of my early trainings and interests; they influenced me to become a psychologist. My third major professional influence was the Enneagram, as conceptualized and taught to me by Don Riso and Russ Hudson.

I wish to pay tribute to the many people who have given me help, support, and encouragement throughout the years: My father, Milton, and mother, Ceil, have given me love and guidance. My brothers Richard and Robert and sisters Lauren and Terri have been a source of support and encouragement. My wife, Jean, has loved and supported me for many years. My daughter, Jamie, has given her unconditional love and encouragement.

In loving memory of my sons, Jason and Jeremy.

Brian S. Grodner, PhD, ABPP, FAClinP

First and foremost, I acknowledge my loving wife, Melissa, whose endless support, encouragement, and personal sacrifice allows me to selfishly pursue my professional endeavors. It is with deep love and admiration that I thank my children, Kailey and Brennan, for their willingness and ability to put aside any immediate requests or needs they had of their father while he was consumed by the demands of this project.

My thanks to David Cox, colleague, advocate, and friend, whose keen attention to detail caught some potentially troublesome typos that other eyes failed to detect.

I'd also like to convey my kindest regards to Phil Laughlin, Senior Editor at Springer Publishing, for his persistent patience and empathic guidance to a freshman author. Future publications will be simpler thanks to his generous assistance.

Finally, I offer my sincerest appreciation to Dr. Brian Grodner, who, due to unfortunate and unforeseen circumstances, was significantly restricted in his ability to actively participate in the creation of this book. I thank him for his willingness to entrust a fellow colleague with completing a text based on his own clinical insights and teachings.

David B. Reid, PsyD

Permanent Habit Control

Practitioner's Guide to Using Hypnosis and Other Alternative Health Strategies

Setting the Stage

PART I

It's choice—not chance—that determines your destiny.

—*Jean Nidetch*

1 Do Old Habits Really Die Hard? Establishing Permanent Habit Control

The best place to find a helping hand is at the end of your arm.

—Swedish Proverb

Throughout this book, you will be offered multiple opportunities to access and mobilize resources, enhance and optimize learning, and maximize use of your time to help yourself and your clients successfully manage unwanted habits. To help prepare for and maximize your learning experience, we encourage you to take a moment and answer the following questions now:

- What are you most motivated and curious to learn and discover? (Think of this in terms of habit control, both personally and professionally.) _____
_____
_____

- What goals would you like to accomplish by learning this material? _____

_____

_____

■ What new skills, attitudes, and feelings do you want to
  manifest? _____

  _____

  _____

■ How do you want to incorporate this new or rekindled knowledge
  into your life on a daily basis in a way that promotes some sense
  of personal growth? _____

  _____

  _____

■ Finally, what are some of your most powerful learning resources?
  (Think in terms of attitudes, skills, beliefs, values, curiosities,
  and capabilities that will support you in accomplishing your habit-
  control outcomes.) _____

  _____

  _____

TEMPORARY CHANGE VERSUS *PERMANENT* CHANGE

If we don't change direction soon, we'll end up where we're going.

—Irwin Corey

Clients seeking help with a variety of concerns, including depression,
anxiety, or panic attacks, to name only a few, frequently request assistance for smoking cessation once they learn this is something we can
help them with. Rather than immediately informing them of our willingness to help them quit smoking, we tell them that our ultimate goal
would be to help them become *permanent* nonsmokers. Notice the subtle
but crucial distinction between their request for help with smoking and
our response to their request. Chances are they've already quit smoking
numerous times before, but were likely unsuccessful in their attempts
at becoming permanent nonsmokers. By informing them that we want
to help them become *permanent* nonsmokers, we set the stage for that
expectation and all that will follow to meet that goal.

As nonsmokers, neither of us would ever consider smoking cigarettes during times of stress. Individuals who quit smoking and yet consider themselves "ex-smokers" maintain personas of people who could once again start smoking under the right (or wrong) circumstances. By starting with the goal of becoming a *permanent* nonsmoker, we help our clients greatly reduce the likelihood that they will ever smoke again. *Permanent* nonsmokers simply *don't* smoke. Period.

This subtle, though seemingly innocuous perspective sets the stage for the expectation that our clients can become permanent nonsmokers. Like Milton Erickson's presupposition technique (see chapter 8), mentioning an intention for our client to become a permanent nonsmoker not only establishes an expectation of success, but immediately initiates relapse prevention.

If a habit-control program like the one offered through this text is to be successful, it is our contention that it must strive to be both positive *and* permanent. By maintaining this supposition, we help people explore the psychology of becoming permanent nonsmokers or permanently slim, fit, and healthy people by telling them the following:

> It's not just what you *do*, it's who you *are*; it's not just your behavior, it's your identity as well. Once change is internalized and integrated, all your positive choices and behaviors become automatic reflections and manifestations of who you are as a permanent nonsmoker. You create a new self-image, a new goal-image of the "new you" having all the attributes and benefits of being a permanent nonsmoker.
>
> We will create a path between the current you and this new you. And by making this image so inviting, so compelling, and so magnetic using special strategies I will teach you, you will move and propel down this path to become this non-smoking "new you." And this new you will guide and direct your behaviors and your choices.

This statement is so important and crucial to the work we do that we encourage you to not only read it again, but commit it to memory or at least use your own words emphasizing the intent of the message. We believe that all behavior, including unhealthy choices like smoking, abusing alcohol, and overeating, have or at least had positive intentions at some point in time in a person's life. It has been our experience that people have healthy intentions to stop smoking, yet remain smokers in their own minds and identities, thereby struggling in a state of continuing inner conflict, tension, and frustration. This of course only enhances the likelihood that they will start smoking again, and most likely sooner than later.

Take David's client Julie, for instance, who once said, "I really want to stop smoking, but sometimes my cigarettes seem to be the only friends I have." Smoking a cigarette at 3 AM when plagued by an unwelcomed bout of insomnia was like calling up a best friend in the midst of a crisis. Sometimes Julie would even talk to her cigarette as she worked it out of the pack, saying things like, "There you are. Come on out of there and spend a little time with me."

For Julie, quitting smoking was like turning her back on a near and dear friend—a friend who had, in her mind, helped her through some very trying times in her life. Her cigarettes were there for her when her husband asked for a divorce, and they were still there for her after she learned he wanted a divorce because he was in love with another woman. They were there for her when she was overlooked for a promotion at work. They were there whenever she needed them.

By offering clients like Julie alternative and equally effective ways to satisfy their positive intentions, you can help ensure they will no longer need to pay the high price of managing life difficulties by smoking and/or overeating. By reducing or resolving stress, negating unwanted urges, and soothing negative emotions that undermine permanent habit control, you will be able to help your clients (or you yourself) become permanent nonsmokers and/or permanently fit and trim individuals. All skills and interventions taught within this book are powerful life-skills that can be applied in any overwhelming and difficult-to-manage life circumstance. While gaining knowledge of and skills for helping your clients learn to become permanently slim and fit or permanent nonsmokers, you will come to see that these valuable skills will always be available, though at times everyone needs a little reminder that these resources are there and available when we need them.

They'll See It When They Believe It: Connecting Your Clients' Everyday Behavior To Their Vision

When it comes to weight loss, the difference between knowing and doing something about the knowing sometimes can be, quite frankly, huge. Finding people who desire to lose weight is an easy task these days. Eavesdrop on a conversation between coworkers in the break room, or on relatives soon after ingesting that second piece of pumpkin pie after Thanksgiving dinner, and you will see that most people readily acknowledge an understanding or at least general knowledge about what is necessary to lose weight. They know they need to cut back on calories, fat grams, and carbohydrates. They can tell you they need to lace up their tennis shoes and take care of business on a stair-stepper or treadmill. Some can even espouse the benefits of an anaerobic training program by incorporating the overload, muscle confusion, and pyramid principles promoted by fitness guru Joe Weider. But finding people who are actually successfully losing weight and keeping it off is a different matter altogether.

Often, people maintain a vision and goal of themselves becoming thin yet continue to engage in self-defeating behaviors (e.g., overeating, sitting around all day, rationalizing that a candy bar, three beers after dinner, or a doughnut won't kill their diet) that contradict their vision of a thinner, healthier body. To implement permanent change, we strive to connect our clients' everyday behavior to their vision.

When establishing and working toward personal goals, desire, though necessary, is insufficient in and of itself. It is not enough to *want* to do something; you must know *how* to do it too. Often, when asking clients to state their goals for therapy, whether it is to be less anxious, less depressed, or simply live a happier life, losing weight generally makes it onto the list. But is stating this desire really enough to accomplish this goal? Aspiration alone won't initiate and maintain the motivation necessary to become permanently fit and trim. After all, sending a man to the moon would have never happened if aspiration hadn't been coupled with good planning, conscious intention, and sustained effort.

Motivational moments, even for people who convincingly verbalize a desire to change, sometimes lack the necessary resources and follow-through to ensure permanent habit control across multiple settings. To live one way at home, yet another at work or elsewhere almost assures failure, not to mention frustration with the inability to become permanently fit and trim. Eating well-balanced weekday meals prepared at home and then feeding like a bottomless pit at the All-U-Can-Eat China Buffet on a Saturday night and indulging in a grand-slam breakfast of sausage, gravy, and biscuits and/or a stack of buckwheat pancakes smothered in butter and syrup the following morning is a diet destined to expand the waistline. The same could be said for the person who eats a healthy dinner only to binge on Rocky Road ice cream and a slice of triple-layered chocolate cake later that night. Such defeatist behavior is analogous to taking one step forward and two back. In many cases, failed diets are only failed because they are not consistently maintained. To become permanently fit and trim, one must maintain persistent consistency between behaviors and desired goals.

Take for instance, Martha, a 62-year-old client David had been working with for several months who was in tears one day because of her failed attempts to lose weight despite doing everything she thought was correct. During the previous 4 weeks, Martha had cut back on her meal portions, started walking nearly every day, was participating in a water aerobics program, and was making healthier food choices, yet *still gaining* weight. The work and sacrifices just didn't seem worth it for her and she was starting to feel hopeless about the possibility that she could ever lose weight. When David asked her to carefully record her weekly diet and document everything that crossed her lips, even if it was a stick of gum, it became readily apparent why Martha was still gaining weight. Although she had indeed cut back on her portions—and though eating smaller portions more frequently through the day is healthier—she had increased her snacking behavior. Despite healthier food choices, Martha was eating more low-fat ice cream and fat-free pastries and cookies late at night. Though low in fat, they were loaded with sugar and carbohydrates. Making matters worse, Martha also reported waking up in the middle of the night several times each night and snacking on peanut butter crackers and Little Debbie's snack cakes. Sometimes she didn't recall doing so, but couldn't dispute the evidence (i.e., food wrappers) found in her bed or scattered about the living room the next morning. And since Martha lived alone, there was no one else to point an accusing finger at when the cookie bin was empty.

So here's a word of caution when helping people become permanently slim and fit: make certain that your clients record *everything* they eat. You may be surprised to find the things that they may not include on the list, believing for some reason that all they need to account for is the food that is consumed for breakfast, lunch, and dinner, and perhaps an occasional snack here or there. Martha is the perfect example of someone who, even unintentionally or subconsciously, neglects to consider late-night snacks or early-morning binges as part of her diet. This certainly underscores the need to use a more formalized, or at least structured, habit history when interviewing clients.

Time management also plays an important role in habit control. In his highly acclaimed (and effective!) book, *The 7 Habits of Highly Effective People,* Dr. Steven Covey emphasizes the importance of learning to "put first things first." Though his book offers numerous suggestions for empowering people to control and manage their lives successfully, one way or the other, the take-home message from Dr. Covey involves wise and judicious management of time. This is readily apparent from the plethora of time-management programs, seminars, personalized daily planners, and PDA devices available for general consumption through his parent company, FranklinCovey.

Though this is by no means an endorsement of FranklinCovey or Stephen Covey himself, it has been our experience and observation that clients tend to limit their success when incongruence exists between their present and their perceived future. When maintaining a cluttered present state of being with hopes and aspirations of empowering a more organized, efficient, and healthier future, people only postpone the change they seek. In essence, the change they desire is eventually buried beneath a pile of other good intentions that failed to come to fruition because the individual lives a cluttered, disorganized life. Learning to manage time and life experiences in the here and now fosters a sense of control and personal mastery over one's destiny and habit control. As Covey says, *begin with the end in mind.* In chapter 6 we explore "timelines" and other activities to critically and objectively evaluate our past, present, and future in ways that encourage and foster lasting change.

When considering behavioral change, whether it is in terms of habit control or improving one's general well-being, many people consciously and perhaps more often subconsciously, place contingencies and limitations on their ability to achieve desired change. Regardless of the goal at hand, people sometimes prematurely sell themselves short by saying things like: "I can be the way I want...*as long as* _____ or *until* _____ or *if only* _____ or *when* _____ or *unless* _____."

Self-imposed and in many ways irrational constraints like these generate unnecessary obstacles that not only impede the initiation of behavioral change, but foster a self-fulfilling prophecy that can spoil any hope for success. By helping clients understand that they can stop smoking or become physically fit *no matter what,* we minimize their tendencies to attach contingencies to a desired goal.

It is with this in mind that we encourage you to tend closely to your clients' language. Listen to not only *what* they say, but *how* they say what they say. By listening to the content *and character* of what they say, you will likely appreciate the limitations they frequently (and subconsciously) place on making healthy changes in their lives. Doing so will allow you to begin to positively influence unconditional change, *no matter what.*

Care for a Snickers Bar?

Think about it for a moment. What difference does a Snickers bar really make? Have you ever picked up a Snickers bar, unwrapped it, and eaten it in a matter of seconds with little concern whatsoever of what it is doing to your body? A 30-pounds-overweight individual could easily look at a Snickers bar or any other unhealthy snack and rationalize, consciously or unconsciously, "Whether I eat this Snickers bar or not, I am still going to be 30 pounds overweight. I'll look in the mirror tomorrow and see no difference. Since it won't make a difference now, I'll eat it and, starting tomorrow, I will go on a diet and watch what I eat."

The *I'll get to it later* perspective only postpones plans to make desired changes in life now and sometimes makes it less likely that the change will ever be initiated. In contrast, maintaining a *no matter what* attitude is not only about behavioral change through time and across contexts, but allows people to recognize that what they do *now* impacts their future self. Permanence requires intentionality. Let's repeat that: *Permanence requires intentionality.* And although we emphasize permanent change throughout this book and in our work with our clients, we certainly do not unconditionally "guarantee" positive results for them or profess that "no further work is necessary" once a desired goal is attained. Rather, we let our clients know that continued awareness and focus in the here and now is essential. Now *and* later.

Robert was 100 pounds overweight and wanted to get back to the athletic, fit Robert that he was before he was married and had two children. He wanted to feel good about himself and his body again. Unfortunately, Robert overate on a regular basis, without much conscious consideration for what his present behavior was doing to his future body. To help him make the connection, Brian had him write a letter to himself as if he were in the future writing a letter to himself in the past. Future Robert wrote a letter to current Robert and sent a message of appreciation to him for the commitments he made to his body and for making healthier decisions that made life better and easier for future Robert.

The benefits of maintaining focused attention and energy in the present can extend to other areas of life as well. Living in the past or projecting oneself into a future of possibilities, particularly if thoughts are riddled with anxiety and worry, only serves to distract us from living our present, here-and-now experience. We tell our clients that the past is nothing more than the wake in the water behind a boat that has no influence on the course the boat is taking. The past never needs to direct our present experience or our future. For many people, however, their past creates an almost certain destiny that restricts and predestines them to an existence over which they perceive little or no control. By the same token, projecting too far into the future, especially if it is anxiety-driven, not only establishes a negative expectation of what may be, but increases the likelihood that the concern or worry will become a reality.

As Dr. Wayne Dyer proclaims in his best selling self-help book, *The Power of Intention,* we can create our own destiny by focusing our intentions on what we really, really, really want. But we must be careful because, if we focus our intentions and energy on what we really, really, really *don't* want (usually that which is based in anxiety, pessimism, and irritability), we just might get that instead. Such pessimism can become infectious and establish a pattern of negative self-fulfilling prophecies.

Perhaps a story will illustrate the point:

One day, a hunter gathered his shotguns, ammunition, and his gifted hunting dog as he headed to his friend's house in preparation for a morning of duck hunting. His friend, a pervasively pessimistic man who could strip the silver lining from any cloud begrudgingly joined him. But the day, contrary to the friend's dour demeanor, was productive. It seemed they couldn't miss a duck if they tried. And one by one, the hunter's faithful dog retrieved each duck, delivering the valued prize to his proud owner. But the dog did so in a rather curious manner. Rather than swim across the lake to retrieve the latest kill, this dog walked on water, with his head held high, duck in mouth, all the way back to the hunters. When the men finally had their fill of hunting, they headed home.

Eventually, the hunter turned to his pessimistic friend and said, "Good day, huh?"

His friend shrugged. "If you say so. A little too cold for my liking."

The hunter ignored the predictable glum reply. "So what'd you think of my dog. Pretty special, isn't he?"

"Special?" the friend snorted. "I don't think so. Your darn dog can't even swim!"

As therapists, it is inevitable that we encounter the perpetual pessimists who for obviously irrational reasons seem to go out of their way to ensure that things just won't or can't work out favorably. They look into their future and "*yeah, but*" and "*what if*" any seasoned therapist to the point that she might be ready to join them by throwing in the towel before the first therapeutic goal is even established. Eventually, a therapist could get to a place where she begins to question, "*What's the point? Why bother?*"

Though clients report a desire to stop smoking or become fit and trim, their pessimistic demeanor can cast doubt on any therapeutic intervention that is intended to offer hope for productive change. But knowing and understanding these clients while helping them focus on the here and now can offer a therapeutic edge when seeking strategic and powerful ways to enhance internal motivation. It is for this and other reasons that we habitually rely on the Enneagram of Personality Types when designing and implementing a treatment plan for our clients. As you will see, having this information at your disposal *before* becoming frustrated with the persistent pessimist (The Loyalist) or distressed with the chronic co-dependent (The Helper) will empower and enable *you* as a therapist to see beyond these apparent detrimental personality traits and work with everything the client brings to treatment, even the "dysfunctional" attitudes and behaviors that keep people stuck and seemingly unable to change for the better.

Just as a healthy permanent relationship with others doesn't leave much room for selfishness when things are going well, neither does establishing a permanent healthy lifestyle. Taking advantage of a healthy relationship (or healthy lifestyle) by acting on selfish motives (or over-eating) almost assures a destructive and dysfunctional relationship (or abandonment of a healthy lifestyle). Consequently, it is important to appreciate and point out to our clients that the notion of "permanent" still requires some continued vigilance to the here and now. There is always work to do if one is to maintain that which is healthy. Losing weight can never be the means to an end. As we often ask our clients, "So let's say you lose 75 pounds through diet and exercise and reach your ideal body weight. Then what?"

Focusing on obtaining and maintaining an ideal body weight through lifestyle change fosters a sense of permanence that is absent when one focuses only on losing a specific amount of weight. For many, failing to appreciate that *permanence requires maintenance* of some kind increases the odds that any dietary program will have a yo-yo effect. Similarly, any well-intended smoking-cessation program that overlooks the need to enhance coping skills will (pardon the pun) be destined to go up in smoke. But it is important to reinforce for our clients that an investment in some goal, whether it is having a successful career, a healthy relationship, or improving one's physical well-being, is always work well worth doing and, eventually, something done willingly. Knowing that the benefits of their efforts to maintain desired behavioral change far outweigh the costs of remaining in a vicious cycle of self-destructive and unhealthy habits, they ultimately remain internally reinforced to keep moving forward.

It has also been our experience that once change is internalized and integrated it is less a matter of vigilance and concentrated effort and more a matter of doing what naturally and spontaneously works.

ADDICTIONS AND THE FOUR C'S

Whereas the term "addiction" does not appear in the most recent version of the *Diagnostic and Statistical Manual of Mental Disorders, Fourth Edition* (American Psychiatric Association, 2000), the term "substance dependence" likely comes closest to capturing the essence of this word. For this reason, we will use the *DSM-IV* Criteria for Substance Dependence as a workable definition of addiction.

Though some believe the term *addiction* should be reserved exclusively for cases involving chemical substances (e.g., Rachlin, 1990; Walker, 1989), we respectfully disagree with this position, as similar diagnostic criteria have been applied to a number of other problem behaviors, including sexual addictions (Knauer, 2002), pathological gambling (Lancelot, 2007), eating disorders (Abraham & Llewellyn-Jones, 2001), video game addiction (Waite, 2007), and technological addiction—which includes Internet addiction (Watters, 2001).

When considering the relationship between habit and addiction, we encourage you to pay attention to The Four C's: compulsion, control, cutting down, and consequence. In many cases, habits will have *compulsive* components to them. When initially evaluating your client, ask yourself, what is the nature of their desire? A compulsion exists when the desire to use something, to ingest something, to *do* something is overwhelming despite other thoughts, feelings, and judgments about the behavior.

It is also important to consider how much *control* the client exhibits over their eating, smoking, or substance use once they have initiated the behavior. Such issues can be very obvious for alcoholics, for whom one drink is never enough. Binge eaters frequently report a lack of control when binging, and this is apparent by how they continue to eat despite becoming physically uncomfortable after gorging themselves with voluminous amounts of food. Likewise, smokers report little conscious regulation of their behavior when lighting one cigarette with the lit end of another, commencing yet another chain of smoked cigarettes.

When addicts and alcoholics *cut down* on their use, adverse effects and unwanted symptoms typically manifest themselves. Therefore, it is important to consider possible withdrawal symptoms that may offer a rough estimate of the extent of an individual's level of dependence on the substance or food.

The following is a list of symptoms suggestive of withdrawal effects associated with dependence:

- Irritability
- Anxiety
- Fatigue
- Insomnia
- Restlessness
- Headache

- Dizziness
- Hypertension
- Excessive sweating
- Nausea and/or vomiting
- Fever
- Rapid heart rate

With either overeating or smoking, cutting down on the unwanted behavior can result in any of the above uncomfortable side effects. At times, these symptoms can initially be mistaken for other emotional concerns and the issues of dependence and withdrawal may be readily overlooked if not considered. About 7 years ago, David had a client he assumed he was treating for severe anxiety and agoraphobia, only to learn after about eight sessions that the symptoms of concern were related to alcohol withdrawal. His client typically arrived to the therapy session complaining of restlessness, insomnia, excessive sweating, and tremulousness. Accordingly, targeted interventions consisted of cognitive-behavioral therapy and progressive muscle relaxation. One day, most unexpectedly, the client presented as if his anxiety had been cured. He displayed no evidence of restlessness, irritability, or anxiety. Within seconds of starting the therapy session, however, it became apparent from the overwhelming stench of stale alcohol in the office that there had been no cure. The gentleman's blood-alcohol level of 0.245 (over three times the legal limit in Virginia) made it glaringly obvious that the presenting symptoms of concern were related to alcohol withdrawal experienced on the day of a scheduled therapy session.

Finally, it is important to consider the *consequences* that continued abuse has on one's physical well-being. Specifically, outright denial despite evidence of physical damage or illness should raise a red flag concerning dependence. Denial by clients takes many forms when their behaviors, whether wanted or unwanted, are questioned or challenged by others. Perhaps your client will tell you "No, my drinking is not a problem; it's fine" when evidence (e.g., history of DUIs, family conflict, public drunkenness charges) suggests otherwise. Or your client may acknowledge the problem but rationalizes or even justifies his behavior by minimizing any ability to control the habit, claiming, "I just can't help myself." Either way, denial of the adverse consequences of behavior or minimization of an ability to change impedes habit control and must be addressed early in the course of treatment if change is to be permanent.

Food as an Addiction

Is there really such a thing as food addiction? Surely you have encountered someone claiming to be a "chocoholic" or perhaps know someone espousing to be "addicted" to certain foods. What about the expectant mother claiming to have "cravings" for certain food, whether it's a slice of New York-style cheesecake or a plateful of Kung Pao chicken? Though food is not technically identified as an addictive substance, an empirical study conducted in 1992 at the University of Michigan School of Public Health addressed this very issue (Drewnowski, Krahn, Demitrack, Nairn, & Gosnell, 1992). Specifically, self-identified "chocolate addicts," when administered the opioid antagonist Naloxone, reported a significant reduction in chocolate and sugar cravings when compared with a placebo control group.

In the 2004 film *Supersize Me*, a documentary offering an irreverent look at obesity in America, filmmaker Morgan Spurlock ate only McDonald's food (breakfast, lunch, and dinner) for 30 days and reported having an addictive-compulsive experience, including variable depressed and elevated mood states associated with fast-food binging. His reported experience is consistent with other addicts who go through withdrawal and relapse during the course of their illness. As an interesting side note, less than 2 months after the film premiered at the Sundance Film Festival, McDonald's announced that it would no longer sell any menu items in "Super Size," though denying their decision was in reaction to the film.

Living in an Obesogenic Culture

Though the number of smokers has declined in most segments of the U.S. population over the past few decades, the same cannot be said of obesity. The prevalence of overweight children and adolescents, and obese men in particular, increased significantly from 1999 to 2004. This trend has not been true of women. However, there were no indications that women were getting any slimmer during this time period;

they just weren't gaining weight to the same degree as their male counterparts or children and adolescents (Ogden et al., 2006). Public health officials believe the alarming increase in morbidly obese people in society has reached such epidemic levels that they now commonly refer to our culture as "obesogenic."

And although the United States has earned its reputation as a country that is literally "bigger than its britches," due in large part to a fast-food mentality in a fast-paced society, it is not alone. Within the last decade, other countries, including Canada, Australia, New Zealand, and Western Europe, have jumped on this unhealthy bandwagon. This, in turn, has fostered other life-threatening and, sad to say, preventable illnesses, including diabetes and cardiovascular diseases (International Diabetes Federation, 2004).

In the not-too-distant past, nearly all children diagnosed with diabetes suffered from the autoimmune form (type I), caused by a diseased pancreas failing to produce adequate levels of insulin. In contrast, type II diabetes, where the pancreas produces normal insulin levels but cells become resistant to it, traditionally took decades to develop. But it seems type II diabetes isn't just for adults anymore. The number of children and adolescents with type II diabetes (most diagnosed in their early teens) has skyrocketed within the last 20 years, prompting the journal *Diabetes Care* to identify it as an "emerging epidemic."

And if it wasn't distressing enough that teens were developing this disease, *Medical News Today* reported, in May 2004, that an obese 5-year-old child weighing 88 pounds in eastern Germany became the youngest child ever to suffer from type II diabetes (Medical News Today, 2004).

Many nonsmokers and fit individuals fail to appreciate the obvious and less obvious ways that obesity and smoking indirectly affect them. Take the airline industry for instance. More recently, when people talk about threats to the airline industry, the primary concern mentioned involves terrorist attacks or threats to our national security. In this instance, though, we are talking about the threat of obesity on the financial stability of major airlines. Through the 1990s, according to the Centers for Disease Control and Prevention, the average weight of Americans increased by 10 pounds. The extra weight caused airlines to spend $275 million to burn 350 million more gallons of fuel in the year 2000 alone, just to carry the additional weight of American passengers. So, as you can see, this epidemic is literally weighing on all of us in very interesting and unusual ways.

Obesity Trends Among U.S. Adults

The Body Mass Index (BMI), a number calculated from a person's weight and height, does not measure a person's body fat directly, yet it is a reliable indicator of "body fatness" and has been shown to correlate with direct measures of body fat, such as underwater weighing and dual-energy X-ray absortiometry (Mei et al., 2002; Garrow and Webster, 1985). Using the BMI as a measurement of obesity, Figure 1.1 shows the body mass trends among American adults from 1990 to 1998 to 2005 to 2007. These figures reflect people who are considered obese and have a BMI of 30 or more. To bring this image to life, a BMI of 30 would be a 5-foot/4-inch person weighing approximately 170 pounds or a 5-foot/10-inch person weighing 207 pounds. A BMI of 25 is considered "overweight" and is reflected in a 5-foot/4-inch individual weighing approximately 145 pounds or a 5-foot/10-inch person weighing 174 pounds.

If you closely examine each state in Figure 1.1, you will clearly see the changes from 1990 to 1998 where what once was light gray, or representative of ideal or healthy BMI, is now darkened to reflect increased BMI. Further, in 2005, fewer states remain within an acceptable BMI range, while a preponderance of states have BMIs above 30 (20 to 24% of the population, with some exceeding 25%).

THE ELUSIVE RELATIONSHIP BETWEEN "HABIT" AND OTHER EMOTIONAL PROBLEMS

Unwanted habits are often an indication that an individual is self-medicating in one form or another. Therefore, whatever concern(s) a client brings to treatment, it is important to consider the relationship between the habit and other emotional problems. As alluded to previously, smoking may be a way of dealing with anxiety, while overeating could be a response to loss, emptiness, or loneliness.

Often, self-medication is a response to trauma and/or other deep-seated emotional issues. It is therefore very important to appreciate that

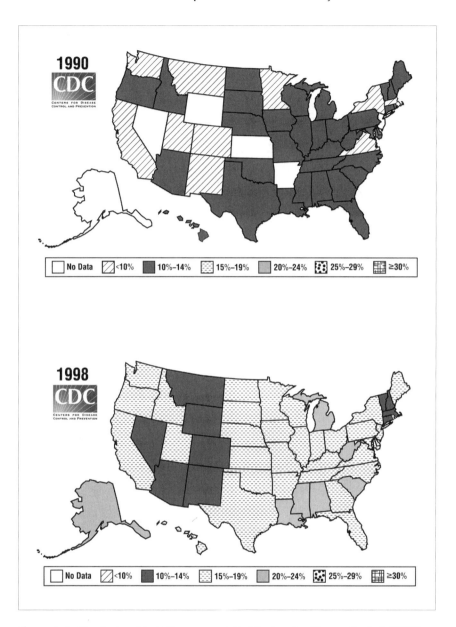

Figure 1.1 Obesity trend in U.S. among adults (Centers for Disease Control, 2007).

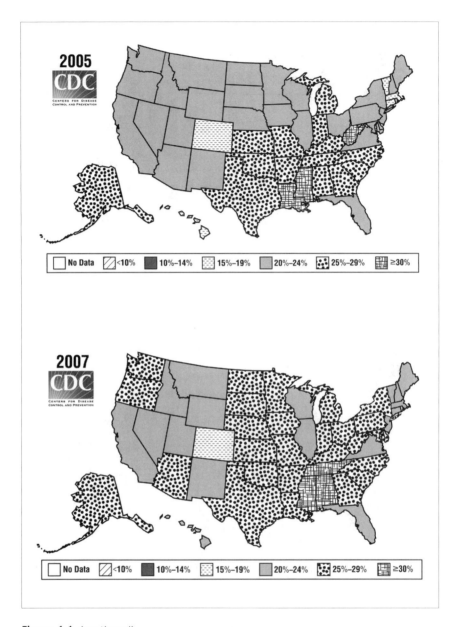

Figure 1.1 (continued)

the desire to lose weight or stop smoking may be more than simply wanting to "kick a habit"; it may have greater psychological significance.

Smoking and Mental Illness

Although smoking among adults has decreased somewhat within the past 10 years, there are still segments of our population, including teenage girls, in which the incidence of smoking is either unchanged or on the rise.

As you most likely know, smokers tend to have a greater rate of depression and other emotional concerns in comparison with control groups. Since chemical and psychological adjustments directly associated with smoking cessation may influence the manifestation of temporary depressive symptoms, it is important to ensure that any client desiring to become a permanent nonsmoker is evaluated and monitored for a mood disorder. Some clients may benefit from psychotropic medication, such as selective serotonin reuptake inhibitors, whereas others could benefit from supportive psychotherapy or a combination of the two.

Interestingly, in a recent article in *Alcoholism, Clinical and Experimental Research,* depression was identified as an important negative predictor of the ability to maintain abstinence from alcohol, whereas depressive symptoms were not significantly related to subsequent abstinence from cigarettes (Kodl, Willenbring, Gravely, Nelson, & Joseph, 2008).

People diagnosed with schizophrenia have significantly elevated rates (45 to 88%) of smoking, compared with people without mental illness (23%). Whereas many clients smoke as a means of controlling stress, anxiety, or depression, recent data suggests that schizophrenics smoke as a means of managing the neuropsychological deficits (e.g., attention, working memory, and thinking and planning) associated with their illness (Dolan et al., 2004).

Preliminary data suggest that schizophrenics have a predisposed vulnerability to nicotine dependence (George et al., 2006); consequently, nicotine replacement therapy is generally essential to minimize physical withdrawal effects and enhance the potential permanence for schizophrenics who smoke. Chantix (varenicline), a partial nicotinic acetylcholine receptor agonist, has received favorable, albeit preliminary support for helping schizophrenics quit smoking (Doggrell, 2007). Whereas most prescriptive medication utilized to help people quit smoking relies on nicotine replacement, Chantix reduces the urge to smoke by blocking nicotine receptors in the brain that in turn trigger the release of a neurotransmitter called dopamine. Since dopamine initiates a fleeting feeling of pleasure, smokers crave this feeling and increase the probability of becoming physically and psychologically dependent on nicotine. Essentially, Chantix blocks nicotine from binding to receptor sites in the brain, thereby preventing the release of dopamine and reducing the urge to engage in behavior (e.g., smoking) that generates feelings of pleasure.

Eating Disorders

Although ours is not a text for treating eating disorders, effective habit control strategies espoused in this book can be readily incorporated into any treatment plan for these syndromes and will be discussed briefly here. As with any initial consultation where eating and weight gain or weight loss is of concern, clinicians should be mindful of the significance of the problem and determine whether it reaches levels of concern typically seen with eating disorders. If you suspect or determine that you client has a serious eating disorder, especially one with dangerous medical implications, additional knowledge and expertise, and perhaps referral for medical consultation, may be necessary before proceeding any further with treatment. In cases like this, we encourage you to consider your profession's ethical code of conduct, as this will likely dictate the course of action that will ensure your client receives appropriate care. At times, however, we have offered consultation to eating disorder specialists, as many of them may not have experience using hypnosis or emotional freedom techniques (EFT) for treating the habit that accompanies other symptoms associated with eating disorders.

Anorexia nervosa, as you may know, is an illness that predominantly affects adolescent girls; however, there has been a rise in the number of boys being diagnosed with the disorder. The most common features of anorexia nervosa include weight loss and a change in behavior in which the weight loss may become severe and ultimately life-threatening. Associated symptoms for females can include dry skin, hypothermia, bradycardia, hypertension, anemia, osteoporosis, cardiac failure, and amenorrhea. Typically, there is an obsessive quality to the person's thinking that is unlikely to be modified by well-intended attempts by concerned friends, family members, and professional health care workers to convince the person that their thinking on the matter is irrational.

You certainly would not expect an individual with anorexia nervosa to arrive at your office seeking assistance to lose weight. She may, however, seek consultation for other habit-related issues, and through the course of treatment you could certainly introduce and encourage alternative and healthier dietary habits using the strategies proposed throughout this book.

Anorexia nervosa can be classified according to one of two primary means involving extreme control: the restrictive type and the binge-eating/purging type.

In the restrictive type, there is no binge eating or purging, simply restriction of food consumption due to an extreme fear of gaining weight. Essentially, individuals diagnosed with restrictive anorexia starve themselves in an effort to gain greater control over their lives, though, in actuality, their extreme behavior ultimately results in serious physical illness and a general lack of control over the body.

Bulimia nervosa, in contrast, involves binge eating, or the consumption of an amount of food that is larger than most people would consume in a specified period of time or circumstance, followed by a purging episode through self-induced vomiting or use of diuretics and/or laxatives. It should be noted that a recent study in the *Journal of Traumatic Stress* confirmed that bulimia nervosa is frequently associated with a history of childhood sexual trauma (Wonderlich et al., 2007). It is therefore prudent to carefully review a client's developmental history to ascertain the possibility of any unresolved childhood sexual abuse.

Whereas most people tend to eat at a certain and typically moderate pace, binge eaters tend to consume their food rapidly. Though such behavior from an outsider's perspective looks like the person is famished, fast-paced eating typically associated with bulimia nervosa has little to do with feeling hungry and more to do with the need to suppress guilt, shame, disgust, and emotional distress. For this reason, binge eating is often done privately and rarely witnessed by others.

At times, a client may not meet all criteria necessary to be diagnosed with either type of eating disorder. The category "Eating Disorder, Not Otherwise Specified (NOS)" characterizes a client who fails to meet specific diagnostic criteria for either of the above-mentioned eating disorders, yet could be classified as suffering from an eating disorder nevertheless. For example, if a woman has all of the symptoms for anorexia nervosa but has a regular menstrual cycle, "Eating Disorder, NOS" would be the appropriate diagnosis.

MOTIVATION: IS IT REALLY ALL THAT?

Motivation has long been considered essential for intentional, permanent behavioral change. Frequently, therapists evaluate their client's motivational level for change during the initial intake meeting. In some instances, therapists may even decline to work with a prospective client if there isn't ample motivation evident to fuel the change. As the saying goes, "You can lead a horse to water, but you can't make him drink."

In their Transtheoretical Model of Behavior Change, Prochaska and DiClemente (1992) identified five stages of readiness for change: precontemplation, contemplation, preparation, action, and maintenance. The premise of this model involves determining a person's current level of motivation and initiating a treatment plan designed to move her to the next level.

Individuals in the precontemplation stage, for instance, have no interest in changing their behavior and tend to close the door on any opportunity for behavioral change. As far as they are concerned, their behavior is perfectly acceptable and there is no need for change. The treatment goal for this individual, therefore, is to motivate him or her in some manner that fosters the likelihood that he or she will consider change, that is, contemplate it. At times, external motivation, either through punishment or uncomfortable consequences for not changing (e.g., incarceration for a DUI; a teenager grounded for not passing classes) or positive reinforcement (e.g., supportive encouragement from 12-step program, family, or friends) moves an individual to the contemplation stage.

Clients in the contemplation stage are considering change, but, at this point, are not doing anything about it. They are hesitant, perhaps because they have tried in the past but failed. Ultimately, they are not ready to commit to change. These are the proverbial window shoppers. As therapists, we want to move contemplators into the preparation phase, where, as you will see, they can begin to anticipate, plan, and put everything in place to initiate change.

Individuals in the preparation stage are at the starting gate. They are planning their change and ready to move forward. They are ready to sign on the dotted line. All they need is a start date and support systems in place to help maintain the change. When an individual is in the preparation stage, the next step is to establish a follow-up plan to facilitate maintenance and minimize relapse. As you will see, this is a very important component of establishing permanent change. For this person, we help them identify themselves as "John, the *permanent* nonsmoker" rather than "John the *ex*-smoker." The former identity assumes that smoking is not a behavioral option for John, whereas the latter to a greater degree clings to the identity of a smoker.

According to DiClemente and Prochaska's model, motivation is essential for change to take place. To quit smoking, the person must first and foremost be motivated to quit. Although there is a certain kind of logic to this line of thinking, it has been our experience that a step-by-step assessment of readiness to change can be somewhat misleading. We believe that people's motivation to change involves more than simply questioning their level of motivation.

It is our contention that one of our roles as therapists is to help clients access, enhance, and actualize their latent and potential motivation. Again, people seek our help because they have not been successful at achieving or maintaining desired change on their own. It stands to reason that perhaps their limited success was in some way related to motivational levels. Why would we take the role of helping with strategies for change, but not apply strategies for enhancing motivation? We agree with DiClemente and Prochaska that motivation is an important element for change, but we also maintain that motivation can be enhanced and activated through well-planned and strategic interventions that extend beyond positive reinforcement or punishment. And although these interventions do not involve pressuring people to do anything against their will, they do help them access resources that may have been overlooked, ignored, or not fully appreciated.

It is also important to realize that motivation is not simply a matter of will power. In fact, for many clients, it is not necessarily "motivation" that provides the foundation for change, but adapting to fear of failure or avoidance of discomfort that maximizes change. When we encounter someone who appears unmotivated, believing they are not ready to change, it is important to realize that their apparent lack of motivation may not be a lack of motivation at all. It may be a matter of fear or anxiety of feeling uncomfortable or concern that they may fail, leaving them little hope that they will ever be able to change. We may have a conversation with them that goes something like this:

"If you knew that you would be successful and you could do it relatively comfortably, would you then want to stop smoking?"

"Oh, yes!" they invariably reply.

"So it's not really a question of your motivation. You *are* motivated. It's just that you had a fear of not being successful, or some concern about feeling uncomfortable. Perhaps if we take care of those concerns for you, your true motivation can help you stop smoking more comfortably and more successfully than you had realized."

HYPNOSIS AND HYPNOTIC LANGUAGE

Throughout this book, we talk about and provide examples of how influential conversational hypnotic language (and hypnosis) can be when woven into the fabric of the entire treatment process. Language is the "mirror of the mind." It shapes and influences (and is shaped and influenced *by*) our experiences, emotions, and internal processing. We use language every day to structure and represent our problems. Therefore, it makes sense to use language to restructure "problem *states*" into solutions, and unwanted reactions into generative behaviors.

Language can be used to facilitate and empower every step of habit control by influencing and directing time and shifting toward movement, possibilities, and positive expectations while steering away from being stuck. Each word or phrase has different meanings and implications. Essentially, nuances in our language are representations of the nuances in our life. When we appreciate that our conversational language is much more literal and less metaphorical than we typically believe, we can begin to understand just how powerful and therapeutic a tool language can be. At the same time, storytelling in therapy, with a carefully measured portion of metaphors, can offer ample motivation that initiates change. For instance, utilization of sports metaphors for the athletically inclined client ("spring training"…"do it for the team" …"step up to the plate") can evoke resources, introduce new possibilities, and fuel the internal motivation necessary to foster productive change (O'Hanlon, 2007).

We will discuss the use of language, intimation, metaphors and other kinds of "extra-communication" throughout this book. As we explore specific treatment strategies, you will, hopefully, begin to appreciate how "hypnotic conversation" can be implemented into nearly every therapy session.

A ROAD MAP FOR INDIVIDUALIZING AND TAILORING THE PROCESS

To help implement permanent change, we want to look and listen, being present in the moment with the client, with a sense of heightened sensory acuity. We need to have our eyes and ears open and attentive while being ever mindful of our client and his reported concerns.

Additionally, we want to utilize our client's belief system, their way of learning, and their perspective and perception when implementing a treatment plan. It is therefore essential to appreciate that the client is a person *first* and a habit/smoker/alcoholic/overeater second. With the advent of specialized treatment, this is an issue that the medical profession continues to grapple with. During David's postdoctoral fellowship at the University of Virginia, it wasn't uncommon for an attending physician to refer to a patient as "*the stroke* in Room 138" or "*the brain injury* just admitted last evening." This dehumanizing classification of people as symptoms or syndromes is something that must be avoided, as it neglects to consider the unique aspects of the person that may be utilized to promote permanent change.

To help keep this perspective in mind, we incorporate the Enneagram of Personality Types into our assessment and treatment of habit disorders. The Enneagram, which we will be discussing in greater detail in chapter 3, is the most practical and profound way to gain personal insight and guidance with clarifying clients' motivation while individualizing and enhancing permanent change. The more familiar you become with this tool, the more empowered you will be to solicit and maintain change—for yourself *and* for your clients.

CONCLUSION

We started this chapter with the consideration that old habits do not have to die hard. We asked you to identify specific goals you would like to establish and accomplish by reading this book and also encouraged you to consider the skills and resources you have available to succeed with the goals you establish. Similarly, by utilizing carefully considered interventions that help clients reframe their perspective and assessment of themselves as being *permanent* nonsmokers and/ or *permanent* slim and fit individuals, we can help them implement behavioral change that fosters *permanent* habit control. It is clear from the empirical research that smoking and obesity generate serious health and environmental concerns that impact all of us, directly and indirectly. Despite this knowledge, and despite massive campaigns designed to help promote healthier behavior, smoking among some groups continues to increase, while obesity is reaching epidemic proportions even among young children. Understanding that unwanted habits at times include positive intentions that challenge the ability to change, we discussed ways to ensure that alternative positive intentions are available and considered, to enhance the likelihood that healthier habits are selected.

Although motivation is strongly correlated with treatment outcome, it is important to understand that motivation alone does not determine the success or failure of treatment interventions. Understanding clients' fears and concerns that impede progress may offer unexplored solutions or resources that could be used to their advantage when initiating a plan for permanent habit control. Similarly, the power of language, and hypnotic language in particular, could be employed in strategic and creative ways to influence a person's readiness to change their unwanted behavior, and to generate the possibility that change will be internalized and permanent.

Things to Do

1. Choose one or two clients or volunteers with habit issues and work with them while reading this book.
2. Choose a personal habit of your own that you would like to treat or improve. This is optional, but highly encouraged so that you may have an opportunity to experience this process firsthand.

3. Be aware of your personal feelings, hopes, concerns, and so on, about treating yourself and others in this context. Keeping a journal of your experiences while reading this book is highly encouraged. This serves as an opportunity not only to communicate your experiences to yourself, but also to monitor your progress and help you remain present-focused, in the here and now.

2 The First Contact

The important thing is to not stop questioning.

—Albert Einstein

In this chapter, we provide a step-by-step approach to understanding your client's present state, history, goals for treatment, and other relevant information that will influence the development and initiation of a treatment plan. In addition to *requesting* information from the client, as you will see, it is important to *suggest* certain information and shape it in ways that help promote success.

GOALS: KEEPING THEM IN THE GAME

Identifying and establishing goals are obviously very important for initiating permanent habit control. Whereas some clients will arrive at your office with no particular goal in mind other than perhaps a general sense of wanting to lose weight, others will identify very specific, concrete goals that they hope to accomplish in therapy. It is important, particularly with this latter group of clients, to help them establish specific treatment goals, as well as establish the criteria—whether conscious or unconscious—that will be used for gauging success.

To this end, we may ask our client, "How will you know that you are successful or that your goals have been met?" From this simple question, we not only determine a client's criteria for success, but also ascertain how well he has (or has not) considered the concern that brought him to our office. At times, and sometimes to our surprise, we learn that his criteria are different from what we might assume them to be. In such instances, it is important to utilize whatever the client brings to the table; however, in due time we may strategically modify his criteria. Initially accepting his ideas permits us to join him in their quest for permanent habit control.

We also want to ask *why now?* Why didn't they call a couple of months ago? Or, to the contrary, why didn't they wait a little while longer before scheduling the appointment? In many cases, there is some precipitating event or some shift in their consciousness that changes their level of motivation. This information is relevant and can be used to help maintain and increase motivation to change.

It is also helpful during the initial interview to be aware of anything that is potentially problematic or, as Brian likes to say, "not ecological." For instance, if a client reports, "I have to stop smoking or my girlfriend is going to leave me," we can be prepared to work with an externally motivating dynamic that may not necessarily elicit permanent change, yet produces initial momentum for change.

THE GENERAL ASSESSMENT

When conducting an intake assessment, it is just as important to have a perspective of the client's overall presentation—her gestalt, if you will—as it is to acquire specific information from her. This not only allows us to understand what the client brings to treatment, but promotes rapport and individualizes treatment planning as well.

Table 2.1 provides a sample of the general assessment considerations we keep in mind while gathering relevant information to promote permanent habit control. Although the questions posed can guide an assessment of your client, you can adapt this assessment to your own needs as well as the needs of your client.

HABIT ASSESSMENT

After the general background assessment is complete and relevant information for tailoring treatment to address the client's needs is obtained,

Table 2.1

GENERAL ASSESSMENT CONSIDERATIONS

Language: What They Say Is How They Think

- What kind of language do the clients use?
- Is there a particular language pattern?
- Do they talk in a very strong, direct, declarative way?
- Do they talk in an equivocal way? We're going to use language to influence them, so we certainly want to know what language they use, because whatever language they use externally, they probably use internally as well.

Attitude: Everybody Has One

- What are their general attitudes?
- Do they tend to be optimistic or pessimistic?
- Do they look at the big picture or focus more on the specific details?
- Do they sort by looking for similarities or for differences?
- What are their overall attitudes toward you, toward therapy, toward life?

Personal Data: Getting to Know Them

- Are they single, married, divorced, or separated?
- Do they have children?
- What is their level of educational attainment?
- Do they live in an urban or rural commmunity?
- What is their income level?
- What is their profession, job, work status?
- What is their ethnicity? There may be ethnic or cultural variables or issues that you want to know about, and that could increase your rapport and positive influence.
- What are their spiritual, religious beliefs? This could provide valuable information that can be used to solicit and enhance motivation for change.

Emotional Status: As You Think, So Shall You Be

- Is there a history of anxiety? Are habits a means of self-medicating?
- Is there a history of depression?
- How are their relationships? Generally supportive? A source of conflict? Argumentative? Sometimes a spouse or partner is not interested in the person changing.
- Do they perceive a lack of control over their habit?
- How do they feel about: their current situation? their health? their physical appearance?
- What are the stressors?
    - Caring for an ill parent, child, or significant other?
    - Do they have other health-related problems?
    - Work?
    - Family?
    - Financial?

we generally turn our attention to a more specific and focused habit assessment.

Most clients are quite capable of describing their current situation, as this is typically what brought them to our office. Nevertheless, at times, clients simply express a desire to quit smoking without providing detailed information concerning their habit. Although such clients may require a more concentrated effort to gather relevant clinical information, this also presents an opportunity to gather specific data about their current situation. Asking questions such as "How much do you smoke?" or "How long have you smoked?" or "When do you smoke?" or "Where do you smoke?" or "Where do you *not* smoke?" will provide a clearer picture of the current status of the person's habit.

After gaining a better understanding of the present situation, we can begin to explore the history of the habit. Asking the following questions will determine the direction and course of the interview:

- How long have you been smoking or overeating?
- When did this habit start?
- Did it start in response to trauma?
- Was it in response to some environmental change or stressor?
- Was it in response to a new relationship?
- Was it influenced by another person?

If, for instance, the habit developed in response to a traumatic event, it would be prudent for the clinician to gather information concerning the dynamics and relationship between the trauma and the unwanted habit. Ultimately, in a case like this, the treatment plan would involve interventions designed to weaken the association between the trauma and the habit. Hypnosis or Emotional Freedom Techniques, in particular, could be utilized to extinguish a more subconscious connection between the trauma and the persistent habit which, over time, has become challenging to undo.

Many habits (healthy and unhealthy) have a longstanding family history predating (and reinforcing) them. Appreciating the negative consequences of unhealthy habits (of which there are likely to be several) should also be explored during the initial interview and revisited from time to time as needed during subsequent treatment sessions. Doing so allows the clinician to reinforce the critical importance of initiating permanent change *now*. For example, if other family members smoke or smoked, it could be helpful to know if any of them suffered from emphysema or died from smoking-related causes. It could also be enlightening to learn how the family responded to the habit and consequences of the habit in an effort to gain a better understanding of the support (or lack thereof) that may be present for the client. Additionally, we would want to know whether the client's habit started in response to a particular family situation and whether other family members developed the habit as well. Perhaps the client started smoking after the death of a loved one, during a contentious divorce, or because of some other family stressor. Therapeutic efforts designed to facilitate the resolution of unfinished family business or help a client adapt to unresolved loss can provide the impetus needed to change behavior.

USING PAST SUCCESSES AND "FAILURES"

Many of life's failures are people who did not realize how close they were to success when they gave up.

—*Thomas Edison*

It is most unusual in clinical practice to encounter people seeking services who have never before tried to lose weight, stop smoking, stop drinking or using drugs, or discontinue whatever the habit or addiction may be prior to their initial appointment. By the time someone comes to you, they have usually tried to change either on their own or with professional assistance, but likely have failed or initially succeeded only to relapse and perhaps regress.

Working with people's successes and failures enhances the probability that they will become permanent nonsmokers and/or permanently fit and healthy. Essentially, we have information (e.g., history) available to us that, at the time the person was trying to change behavior, was not available to them. It is therefore important to access this information and ask about other attempts at habit control.

Learning what did and did not work for the client enhances future habit control success. The following questions serve as a guide for gathering this most beneficial data:

- Have you ever stopped smoking?
- How long did you stop smoking?
- What happened for you to start smoking again?
- Has there been a time when you lost weight intentionally?
- How much weight did you lose?
- How long did you keep the weight off?
- What was helpful before? What worked?
- What didn't work?
- Were there any downsides to losing weight?
- What happened for your successes and progress to discontinue?
- What were you thinking the moment you decided to smoke again or consume unhealthy meals?

Of course, we want to explore factors that enhanced success as well. Understanding what worked for an individual and how she or he implemented successful interventions to promote habit change can and should be capitalized upon. In particular, we want to understand what was and wasn't helpful, so as not to reinvent the proverbial wheel. Knowing what worked in the past may allow us to re-implement past successes in a new context now, which could make the difference between temporary and permanent habit change.

Though at first glance it may seem counterintuitive, clinicians should consider any possible negative ramifications of success. For example, someone may have lost weight, but sibling jealously may have impeded continued success. Or perhaps weight loss generated insecurity in an unsupportive spouse, who sabotages any weight loss efforts by buying fattening foods. So, it is possible to have successes meet with resistance that challenges progress and creates instability in the greater ecology of the person.

Because something happened in the person's life for progress to cease—otherwise, he or she would not be seeking your assistance—we also gather information about the termination of success. Brian once worked with a young woman who succeeded in stopping smoking, and did so for many years until she bought a pack of cigarettes and relapsed. When he asked why she didn't just do what she had done in the past to stop from smoking, she told him her inner conflict at the time overwhelmed any willpower she needed to not smoke. One cigarette led to the next and before she knew it, she was up from a pack to a pack-and-a-half a day. In the end, she decided it wasn't worth the effort to quit the way she did before, given the price she thought she would have to pay because it was so uncomfortable for her to quit the first time. Essentially, she told Brian that if she was going to quit smoking again, she needed to do it in a way that was more comfortable. Thanks to this information, Brian was able to design a treatment plan that relied upon her past successes in a way that was more comfortable for her.

Asking the question, "What happened? What did you say to yourself right before you smoked that first cigarette?" may elicit helpful information to help a person quit smoking. Perhaps the client tells you she said, "Ah, to hell with it, I am so upset I might as well smoke" or, "One will not hurt, I want to test myself anyway"?

We then ask the client to take a sheet of paper and divide it in half. On the left side of the paper we have him write down any internal dialogue that was occurring just before having that first cigarette. Sometimes the voice he recognizes is a younger, pleading, whiney, or belligerent addictive voice. Perhaps he is using "junko" logic to justify smoking, the kind we would never accept from an oppositional or defiant child who may say, "I had a rough day, I deserve to shoplift." Clients, as we are sure you have observed at some point in your experience, readily accept this kind of justification or rationalization from themselves.

On the right side of the paper, we encourage the client to provide a more objective reaction to her rationale for smoking. It may go something like this: "One *will* hurt, I could get cancer" or "I had a hard day, and maybe I feel like I deserve a cigarette—but what I really deserve is a nap, or some peace and quiet reading a book." We encourage the client to challenge the irrational thinking that reinforced the unwanted behavior, in much the same way a cognitive-behavioral therapist would assist a depressed client to reconsider the automatic, irrational beliefs that have been maintained over time that foster persistent depressive experiences. For instance, if our smoking client wants to test herself, instead of smoking a cigarette, we may have her identify healthier tests or challenges she can undertake. Perhaps she can go for a walk, or hike through the woods, or engage in some friendly competition with a significant other—preferably an activity that requires at least moderate physical exertion.

Ultimately, if we understand the nature and circumstances of when and how a client relapses, we can proactively initiate a plan to ensure that there is an intervention in place that minimizes the possibility of a relapse. This way, we implement preemptive relapse prevention.

Knowing what wasn't effective in the past can be just as important to our intervention as knowing what worked, but didn't last. Although initiating a previously ineffective treatment plan is pointless, it may make sense to adjust a person's past experience to a degree that a new situation is different enough to enhance success. This will become particularly relevant when using hypnosis in creative and strategic ways to access and mobilize frequently untapped resources that facilitate change.

HABIT CONTROL RESOURCES

Everyone has resources or personal life experiences at his or her disposal that can facilitate positive change in the course of his or her life. Though some of us may be more skillful at accessing and employing these resources, all of us possess them nonetheless. Helping clients identify and use personal habit control resources can be a very empowering experience, for them and for us. To help initiate momentum in this regard, we inquire about the client's general beliefs concerning change and his or her perspective about life in general. How does she think things occur and change in the world? What are her religious or spiritual beliefs? Are her attitudes about change generally optimistic or pessimistic? Is the glass half full, or half empty? Either way, as previously mentioned, we will work with whatever the client brings to help influence change.

Though some clients immediately minimize or deny possessing sources of support in their lives, believing themselves to be alone in their struggles, direct questioning may yield previously unrecognized assistance that can be used in their habit control plan. These may include family, friends, supervisors, coworkers, counselors, ministers, and so on. By asking the right questions, we may learn of certain skills our client has in one area of his life that would be very powerful and effective if transferred and applied to his or her habit control issues. Perhaps he has had experiences in which he had to rely on perseverance, or the ability to focus in an effort to overcome odds. Maybe at some time in his life the client implemented certain strategies to give up alcohol or drugs but are not employing them now to stop smoking or initiate a healthy diet and weight loss plan. David typically asks his clients what their greatest accomplishment or proudest moment has been thus far in their life. Focusing on a history of positive results will set the stage for solutions far better than examining the reasons why certain interventions just won't work. The latter mindset establishes expectations of failure and pessimism whereas attention directed on the former fosters a sense of solution-oriented success.

As we work with our clients, we also want to have a general understanding of their knowledge level and social sophistication. This data is very beneficial for guiding and individualizing treatment, as it helps determine not only how much information should be shared with a client, but *how* that information should be shared. For instance, in some cases, professional jargon that is unfamiliar to the general public should generally be avoided. It has been our experience that using jargon tends to distance some people from treatment and can inhibit the development of therapeutic rapport and trust.

LOCUS OF CONTROL

Julian Rotter introduced the term *locus of control* in his Social Learning Theory (1966), which refers to a person's belief about the main causes of certain events in his or her life. Rotter proposed that people maintain general beliefs and opinions about what determines whether or not they will receive reinforcements in life. He classified people along a continuum from very internal (believing success or failure is largely within their control) to very external (believing reinforcements in life are the result of luck, chance, or powerful people). In other words, "internals" attribute success or failure to themselves and "externals" see little impact of their own efforts on the amount of reinforcement they receive. Locus of control is a generalized expectancy that to some extent can predict people's behavior across contexts; however, Rotter made it clear that there are specific situations where externals may engage in behaviors more reflective of internals and vice versa.

Though the process of identifying a client's locus of control may seem unnecessary, it can influence how direct, how authoritarian, how permissive, and how active our interventions will be. For instance, we want to know the client's general sense of personal responsibility. Does she believe the current situation is based on what she is doing, or does it seem beyond her direct level of control? Does she have a sense of empowerment that success (or lack thereof) is in her own hands and dependent on her own actions? Or does she perceive the situation to be the responsibility of her family, friends, or perhaps bad luck? Externals, for instance, tend to be dependent types, seeking a quick fix, a zap, a diet that takes care of every meal, every challenge. Externals can also be unduly influenced by environmental cues and triggers that may be so tempting and influential that they can't believe they lack control over their behaviors. When it comes to treatment interventions, individuals who have an external locus of control tend to expect change to occur because of what the therapist does, not because of what they themselves do. Perhaps a case example will better illustrate the dynamics:

> Sylvia was a 58-year-old female seeking assistance for smoking cessation. She consented to hypnosis after David provided her with all necessary and relevant information to proceed with treatment. She reported smoking two to three packs of cigarettes per day for the past 30 years and met all criteria for nicotine dependence. She smoked her first cigarette of the day immediately upon awakening and had her last cigarette of the day immediately before retiring to bed. She smoked when feeling ill, and chain smoked throughout the day. As the initial interview was coming to a close, she asked, "So when are you going to hypnotize me so I can stop smoking?" David explained the typical treatment protocol, including an estimated number of sessions to help Sylvia stop smoking, and she was shocked and dismayed that it wasn't a "one-time thing" that magically warded off any subsequent desire to smoke. Her expectation of a "quick fix," with little responsibility or accountability on her own part, clearly indicated that she was an individual with an external locus of control. Unfortunately, she was an extreme external, who failed to schedule a follow-up appointment as she had hoped that David could put her in a trance, offer a suggestion or two, snap his fingers to bring her out of trance, and send her on her way to become a permanent nonsmoker forevermore.

Sylvia is obviously an example of an extreme case of someone with an external locus of control, but this does underscore the importance of understanding a client's perspective on change, which clearly influences the course of treatment. In this particular case the course of treatment ended before it could begin.

In an effort to identify someone's locus of control, we would question how much he attributes his level of control over smoking, weight, drinking, drug use, or whatever habit or addiction he desires to change.

Table 2.2

DETRIMENTS FROM CHANGE VERSUS NO CHANGE

	CHANGE	NO CHANGE
Me	Harold might get jealous. My friends may not like me. Pressure to keep weight off and exercise.	Feel bad about myself. No new clothes. Stay tired all the time.
Harold	May get jealous. Think other men are attracted to me. I will have to spend money on new clothes.	Tell me I'm "fat," Give me a hard time for what I eat.

We also question how much accountability for change is placed on his behavior and responsibilities versus external factors that seem beyond his control.

CHANGE VERSUS NO CHANGE

Is it really in the client's best interest to change? This may seem like a strange question to ask, but by reviewing with our clients the pros and cons of changing versus not changing, we may influence a decision and enhance an individual's motivation to change.

Most conscious decisions to change behavior involve some sense of cognitive dissonance or discomfort. Otherwise, implementing change would be a simple matter requiring little to no assistance or support from others. Consequently, we believe it is important to examine the detriments to the client and others in the client's life that may accrue from making the change and the detriments to the client and others in the client's life that may accrue from *not* making the change.

We use the two-by-two grid in Table 2.2 to explore this information with our clients. As you can see, it has been filled in, using information obtained from one of David's clients who was seeking services for weight management. The client was a 33-year-old married female who provided information concerning the detriments that she perceived would accrue, both to herself and to her husband, if she were to lose weight.

These four categories can provide relevant insight into a client's internal dynamics and external behaviors. In this case, it is apparent that David's client has concerns about how her husband will react to her losing weight. It is therefore important to perhaps include him in her treatment, either directly by inviting him in for a session, or indirectly by having the client speak to her husband about her concerns. Either way, if the client maintains these concerns about her husband's reactions, yet doesn't address them during treatment, she is almost assured that losing weight will involve an ongoing battle that may or may not be necessary. In this particular case, David encouraged his client to share her concerns with her husband and, after doing so, she found that he was far more supportive of her losing weight than she had imagined. After soliciting his support, he too became motivated to lose weight and become permanently fit. They became great supports for each other and the concerns she had about his jealousy of her new body and her need to purchase new clothes disappeared.

We revisit this important issue when we focus specifically on the reasons to change and the reasons to maintain the status quo.

NICOTINE ADDICTION SCREENING (FAGERSTROM–RUSTIN)

Cigarette smoking involves both psychological and physically addictive reactions to nicotine. We have generally noted that the psychological habit in particular is the stronger influence and has the greatest impact upon smoking behavior. If smoking were predominantly a physically addictive matter, nicotine replacement therapy (NRT) alone would be much more effective for smoking cessation.

Nonetheless, it is important to estimate the relative physical addictive nature of a client's smoking so that we can estimate the level of nicotine dependence and potential withdrawal effects that may challenge and perhaps impede an individual from becoming a permanent nonsmoker.

The Fagerstrom Test for Nicotine Dependence (Heatherton, Kozlowski, Frecker, & Fagerstrom, 1991) is an easy-to-administer and helpful questionnaire that can determine the need for NRT (see Table 2.3). It is important to keep in mind that these questions simply identify

Table 2.3

FAGERSTROM TEST FOR NICOTINE DEPENDENCE

	0 POINTS	1 POINT	2 POINTS	3 POINTS
How soon after you wake up do you smoke your first cigarette?	>60 min	31–60 min	6–30 min	<5 min
Do you find it difficult to refrain from smoking in places where it is forbidden (e.g., church, library, cinema?)	No	Yes		
Which cigarette would you hate most to give up?	Any other	First one in the morning		
How many cigarettes per day do you smoke?	<10	11–20	21–30	>30
Do you smoke more frequently during the first hours of waking than during the rest of the day?	No	Yes		
Do you still smoke if you are so ill that you are in bed most of the day?	No	Yes		

Classification of dependence:
0–2	very low
3–4	low
5	moderate
6–7	high
8–10	very high

Note: From Heatherton, Kozlowski, Frecker, and Fagerstrom (1991). Reprinted by permission.

probabilities, not clear, consistent correlations between behavior and nicotine dependence. For instance, whereas one question, "How many cigarettes do you smoke per day?" generally reflects a level of nicotine dependence, some clients who smoke less than one pack per day may have a higher level of nicotine addiction than clients who smoke more, simply because of their strong psychological needs and habits.

Nicotine dependence is enhanced if an individual smokes first thing in the morning, either in bed or as soon as he gets out of bed after landing his feet on the floor. If the client waits 30 minutes or an hour, has breakfast, or takes a shower before smoking the first cigarette of the day, then there is relatively less physical addiction.

The most important cigarette of the day can offer insight into the probability of physical dependence and the need for supplementation. If a client can "give up" that first cigarette of the day as if it weren't that important, nicotine replacement becomes less necessary. On the other hand, if a client just can't get going until she has had that first cigarette, the likelihood of dependence and need for some means of supplementation is increased. We also like to ask our clients what's most important: smoking the first cigarette or having the first cup of coffee of the day. Many clients have difficulty selecting one over the other because the two are often paired together for most smokers; however, when the cigarette is chosen over the coffee, our clients typically have very high dependence ratings as identified on the Fagerstrom Test for Nicotine Dependence.

Determining what happens if an individual can't smoke offers insight into his behavioral reactions when his ability to engage in the habit is restricted. For instance, if he was on an airplane, in school, at work, or in some other public facility or environment that prohibits smoking, how would he react? What would he do? Would the client adapt without problem, or become antsy and agitated to the degree that he would sneak a few drags off a cigarette regardless of the potential consequences. Obviously, the latter situation bodes more poorly for nicotine dependence. The same holds true for the individual who smokes during an illness, and this question serves as the fifth and final question on the Fagerstrom Test for Nicotine Dependence.

Scoring the Fagerstrom is pretty simple and straightforward. As stated earlier, the final score offers a probability for physical dependence and should not be used as an absolute score to determine if someone should or should not utilize NRT. Some clients whose scores fall in the low to moderate range (e.g., 3 to 5) may initially wish to forego replacement therapy and reconsider it if they experience physical discomfort from having stopped smoking.

Nicotine-Replacement Therapy

The majority of our clients who wish to stop smoking do not use NRT. In fact, most people do not require nicotine replacement and some, if they used some supplementation, may end up increasing their exposure to nicotine more than when they were smoking. If, however, a client appears to have what we refer to as a *high loading* of physical addiction, we generally encourage this person to seek some means of nicotine replacement or alternative smoking cessation medication. At times clients arrive with the expectation that NRT is essential and they wouldn't consider quitting smoking without this aid. If after completing a thorough assessment and having the client complete the Fagerstrom Test for Nicotine Dependence it seems most likely that the client is physically dependent on nicotine and likely to experience very uncomfortable withdrawal symptoms, then we discuss with her the options available for minimizing physical discomfort as she quits smoking. There are many options for nicotine replacement, including gum, patches, lozenges, and nasal sprays. Of course, it is essential for clients to consult with their physicians prior to initiating any NRT (even over-the-counter products), as there are associated adverse side effects and interactive effects that may preclude someone from using nicotine supplementation.

Nicotine Patch

The nicotine patch releases a constant amount of nicotine in the body. Unlike the nicotine in tobacco smoke, which passes almost instantaneously into the blood through the lining of the lungs, nicotine in the patch can take up to 3 hours to pass through the layers of skin and into the blood stream. Patches are similar to adhesive bandages and are available in different shapes and sizes. The patch is generally worn all day and is not to be put on and removed as a substitute for having a cigarette. Most of the patch products are changed once every 24 hours, though one particular patch is worn only during the waking hours. Wearing the nicotine patch lessens chances of suffering from several of the major smoking withdrawal symptoms, such as tenseness, irritability, drowsiness, and lack of concentration, though there are some side effects, including skin irritation, dizziness, racing heartbeat, insomnia, headache, vomiting, muscle aches and stiffness, and nausea.

Incidentals. It is important to change locations on the body when applying a new patch, as it can cause irritation and minor burning. Some have reported very vivid dreams when the patch is applied late in the evening, before bedtime. To avoid or minimize vivid dreams, the patch can be applied earlier in the day or removed while sleeping. The average retail price for over-the-counter transdermal nicotine patches (starter box) is approximately $4.00 to $5.00 a day.

Nicotine Gum

Nicotine gum delivers nicotine to the brain more quickly than the patch; however, unlike cigarette smoke, which passes almost instantaneously into the blood through the lining of the lungs, the nicotine in the gum takes several minutes to reach the brain. This makes the "hit" with nicotine gum less intense than with a cigarette. Nicotine gum is not designed to be chewed like normal gum, but rather used in the "chew and park" method. After inserting the gum into the mouth, it is to be chewed a few times to break it down, after which time it's parked between the gum and cheek and left there. The nicotine from the gum will make its way into the body via the blood vessels just under the lining of the oral cavity. If chewed instead of parked, the nicotine will be released directly into the saliva, which will eventually be swallowed, causing a very uncomfortable stomachache as well as cravings for a cigarette.

Nicotine gum contains enough nicotine to reduce the urge to smoke. The over-the-counter gum is available in 2-mg doses (for smokers of 24 or fewer cigarettes each day) and 4-mg doses (for smokers of 25 or more cigarettes each day). One piece of gum is one dose; maximum dosage should not exceed 24 pieces per day. Empirical studies have shown that nicotine gum helps take the edge off cigarette cravings without providing the tars and poisonous gases found in cigarettes and is a temporary aid that reduces symptoms of nicotine withdrawal after quitting smoking (Silagy, Lancaster, Stead, Mant, & Fowler, 2002).

Incidentals. Nicotine gum comes in several different flavors, including mint and fruit. Nicotine gum is not advised for individuals with temporomandibular joint disorder (TMJ), as it could promote additional pain and discomfort. Hiccups are a common side effect when the gum is consumed or chewed too quickly. The average retail price for nicotine gum is approximately $4.50 a day (10 pieces) for average usage during the first 6 weeks.

Nicotine Lozenge

In 2002, the first and only over-the-counter nicotine lozenge meant to help smokers kick the habit was made available for public consumption. Nicotine lozenge comes in the form of a hard candy and releases nicotine as it slowly dissolves in the mouth. Eventually, the quitter will use fewer and fewer lozenges during the 12-week program until he is completely nicotine-free. Biting or chewing the lozenge will cause more nicotine to be swallowed quickly and result in indigestion and/or heartburn and results in less efficacy. Nicotine lozenge is available in 2-mg or 4-mg doses. One lozenge is one dose and the maximum dosage should not exceed 20 lozenges per day.

Incidentals. Lozenges tend to become "slimy," producing an odd texture and consistency that can be unpleasant and easy to accidentally swallow. If the individual is prone to dry mouth, a chalky-white buildup can develop at the sides of the mouth, creating a potentially socially embarrassing experience. The most common side effects of lozenge use include soreness of the teeth and gums, indigestion, and throat irritation. Each lozenge will last about 20 to 30 minutes and nicotine will continue to leach through the lining of the mouth for a short time after the lozenge has dissolved. The average retail price for nicotine lozenge is approximately $6.00 a day for average usage (12 doses) and up to $12.00 a day for maximum usage (20 doses) during the first six weeks of use.

Nicotine Spray

Nicotine nasal spray, dispensed from a pump bottle similar to over-the-counter decongestant sprays, relieves cravings for a cigarette and is available only by prescription. Nicotine is rapidly absorbed through the nasal membranes and reaches the bloodstream faster than with any other NRT product, giving a rapid nicotine "hit" which makes it attractive to some highly dependent smokers. The most common side effects of the nasal spray are nose and throat irritations. A usual single dose is two sprays, one in each nostril. The maximum recommended dose is five doses per hour or 40 doses total per day.

Incidentals. Nicotine nasal spray bottles should remain out of reach of children, as they have toxins that can be fatal to young children and animals. The average retail price for nicotine nasal spray is approximately $5.00 a day for average use (13 doses) and up to $15 a day for maximum usage (40 doses).

Nicotine Inhaler

The nicotine inhaler, also available only by prescription, consists of a plastic cylinder containing a cartridge that delivers nicotine when "puffed." It is used only during cigarette cravings and should not exceed more than 16 cartridges a day for up to 12 weeks. Although similar in appearance to a cigarette, the inhaler delivers nicotine into the mouth, not the lung, and enters the body much more slowly than the nicotine in cigarettes.

Each cartridge delivers up to 400 puffs of nicotine vapor. It takes at least 80 puffs to obtain the equivalent amount of nicotine delivered by one cigarette. The initial dosage is individualized and the best effect is achieved by frequent, continuous puffing for 20 minutes. One cartridge will last for 20 minutes of continuous puffing and deliver 4 mg of nicotine; only 2 mg of which are actually absorbed. This is the equivalent of about two cigarettes.

Side effects of the inhaler include irritation of the throat and mouth, usually after the first few uses.

Incidentals. Inhalers work much quicker than gum and also resemble cigarettes to give the user the "feeling" of smoking. In the end, however, the device may prolong the time it takes to quit, as it mimics the physical behaviors of smoking that eventually must be extinguished. Inhalers require daily cleaning and, like nasal sprays, cartridges should remain unopened until needed, as they have toxins that can be fatal to young children and animals. The average retail cost of the nicotine inhaler is approximately $45.00 for a package (42 cartridges) and is generally not covered by most health care insurance policies.

Medications

Zyban (buproprion hydrochloride), which is the antidepressant Welbutrin, appears to help clients who start it 1 week or so before giving up cigarettes completely. One of the reasons Zyban may work better than other antidepressants is the heavy uploading of dopamine and, to some extent, norepinephrine. Dopamine is considered the reward neurotransmitter and cigarettes as well as many other addictions seem to involve dopaminergic centers of the brain.

Common side effects include insomnia, dry mouth, and dizziness. Treatment with Zyban begins while the user is still smoking, 1 week prior to the quit date. Treatment is then continued for 7 to 12 weeks, though length of treatment tends to be individualized.

The average wholesale price for Zyban is approximately $2 per day and in most cases is covered through medical insurance companies.

The newest prescription drug, Chantix (varenicline tartrate), is only the second nicotine-free smoking-cessation drug to gain FDA approval. The active ingredient varenicline works in two ways: by cutting the pleasure of smoking and by reducing the withdrawal symptoms that lead smokers to light up again and again.

The tablet is taken twice daily for 12 weeks, a period that can be doubled in patients who successfully quit, to increase the likelihood they remain smoke-free.

Common adverse side effects include nausea, headache, vomiting, gastric distress, insomnia, abnormal dreams, and a change in taste perception.

In our opinion, nicotine therapy is beneficial in some cases, though not the most effective or efficient intervention for smoking cessation. When using nicotine therapy alone, individuals do not address the other important issues that accompany smoking and smoking cessation and so extend the process of change.

CREATING A PROPULSION SYSTEM FOR CHANGE AND EMPOWERING PROGRESS

There are two major categories of motivation, *moving towards* motivation and *moving away from* motivation. Moving away from pain or moving away from what you do not want is a means of motivation. The other kind of motivation involves moving towards something, usually some identified goal. For instance, moving toward pleasure, a desired outcome, or some positive reinforcement, involves motivation toward progress. Although one may seem more inviting than the other, it is important that we use both when working with our clients.

We have a tendency to use more *moving away from* pain or displeasure motivation; however, the more we use *moving away from* motivation, the more fear becomes part of the process. Perhaps an example will help illustrate this.

If a client is 20 pounds overweight and upset with his weight and begins to gain more weight, he is likely to become even more distressed. Suppose he gains another 20 pounds and now he is so upset that he finally decides to do something about it by initiating a healthy diet and exercising. Because the weight gain enhanced his level of motivation to initiate some plan, what happens to his level of motivation as he begin to lose weight and gets closer to his desired weight? Will he lose motivation now that he doesn't have much more weight to lose? Will he be motivated to continue with his program once there is no more weight to lose? Will maintaining be enough? Perhaps therein lies the root of the "yo-yo" weight loss–weight gain experience.

When you use moving-away-from motivation (i.e., moving away from what you fear), the closer you are to your goal the less the motivation: "Now I am only 28 pounds overweight and my motivation to change is not as great as it was when I was 40 pounds overweight."

On the other hand, if I use moving-toward motivation (i.e., moving toward what I want), the closer I am to obtaining my goal the more motivated I am to continue to pursue it. It is like a runner approaching the finish line, giving it all he has on the final lap.

We do not want to exclusively employ moving-toward motivation when working with a client, as this is not very practical. For example, using only moving-toward motivation may mean we decide not to wear seatbelts or not brush our teeth or perhaps be inclined to driving around mountain curves at 80 miles/hours because it is exciting and there is no fear at all. A blending of the two kinds of motivation tends to be most beneficial for most clients, though in general the ultimate goal is to enhance a level of internal motivation that generates lifestyle changes and enhances permanent habit control.

Our objective is for motivation to operate as a propulsion system. Pushing away from what the client doesn't want (e.g., emphysema, being uncomfortable on an airplane) and being pulled toward what the client desires (e.g., more energy and looking better). This propulsion system, incorporating both kinds of motivation, is empowering and offers greater utility than either moving towards a desired goal or moving away from an unwanted fear.

CONCLUSION

In this chapter we provided a step-by-step approach to understanding your client's present state, history, goals for treatment, and other relevant information that influences the development and initiation of a treatment plan. In addition to *requesting* information from the client, we reviewed the importance of making *suggestions* to our clients that influence and promote success as well as gaining a greater understanding of past successes and failures concerning habit change.

As part of the initial evaluation, which provides the foundation for the treatment plan, we acquire information about the benefits of changing versus not changing behavior in addition to evaluating our client's supports, internal and external resources, and locus of control as determined by the Rotter Locus of Control Scale, a self-administered forced-choice questionnaire.

More specifically, we focused attention on smoking cessation and the need to determine the necessity of NRT or other medical interventions designed to curb cravings and facilitate smoking cessation. Finally, we reviewed pragmatic strategies for facilitating a propulsion system for empowering change.

Things to Do

1. Practice taking at least one habit-control history of a client who expresses a desire to quit smoking or lose weight.
2. Administer and score the Locus of Control Scale for several clients and for yourself. Incorporate the results of this test into a treatment plan that fosters permanent habit control.

3 The Enneagram*

He who knows others is learned. He who knows himself is wise.

—Lao Tzu

INTRODUCTION

The Enneagram (pronounced ANY-a-gram) is a profound yet practical method for understanding ourselves and those who are important in our lives. When used properly, the Enneagram helps us appreciate why we have conflicts with certain people, while with others we may feel an instant and perhaps longstanding bond or connectedness despite knowing them for only a brief period of time. In addition to enlightening us about our own personalities, the Enneagram has also proven to be very beneficial for enhancing relationships, facilitating conflict resolutions, and fostering an individual's personal growth.

*The authors gratefully acknowledge and appreciate Don Russo and Russ Hudson for their insight and understanding as well as the development of the Enneagram. Most of the descriptions of the Enneagram system and types in this chapter are restatements of the work and teachings of Don Riso and Ross Hudson, combined with our application of their mateiral to habit control issues and treatment.

Although the Enneagram is best known as a psychological and spiritual tool, it is also very practical for business applications, including effective and efficient management of personnel, employee motivation and productivity, and ultimately improved company profitability. For the purpose of this book, the Enneagram will be employed to gain a greater understanding of our clients and their personalities so that a more individualized and strategically tailored treatment plan can be developed and implemented in ways that enhance permanent habit control.

WHAT IS THE ENNEAGRAM?

Before delving into the specifics of this fascinating tool, let's first consider the history of the Enneagram, and how we have come to understand and implement the very pragmatic data it provides.

The Enneagram is a geometric figure that delineates nine basic human personality types and their complex interrelationships. Each of the nine types has its own set of perceptions and preoccupations, values, and understanding of and approaches to life. No one type is better or worse than the other, and although the Enneagram symbol suggests that there are nine basic personality types, there are, of course, several subtypes and variations within these nine primary categories. Unlike many personality typologies or objective personality tests you may be familiar with, it is not the intention of the Enneagram to place an individual in a box, or reduce a person's complex personality to one simple category. And though many in the behavioral health field are well acquainted with pathology-based personality inventories whose primary objective is to rule out or rule in certain diagnostic possibilities (e.g., narcissist, passive-dependent, or antisocial personalities), the Enneagram is a tool that helps understand the human personality and overall patterns in human behavior, including inherent strengths and abilities as well as deficiencies and abnormalities.

As a symbol, The Enneagram is a modern synthesis of a number of ancient wisdom traditions that was first brought to the attention of the modern world by the Greek-Armenian mystic George Invanovitch Gurdjieff around the turn of the 20th century. The Enneagram symbol has roots in antiquity and has been traced back to the works of Pythagoras. The typology now associated with the symbol was initially developed by Oscar Ichazo. Ichazo was the founder of the Arica school of self-realization and, in developing the basic principles of Enneagram theory, borrowed heavily from classic Greek philosophy and ancient spiritual ideas from mystical Judaism and early Christianity. While living in South America, a group of Americans, including noted gestalt psychiatrist and anthropologist Dr. Claudio Naranjo and mind/brain researcher Dr. John Lilly (best known for inspiring the film *Altered States*), went to Arica, Chile, to study with Ichazo to gain a greater understanding of the methods he proposed for attaining self-realization. The group spent several weeks with Ichazo, learning the basics of his system and applying the seminal practices he taught them.

Impressed with the system espoused by Ichazo, Dr. Naranjo brought the Enneagram to the United States and, within a few years, this powerful typology gained recognition throughout North America. Within a few years, Don Riso began exploring and studying the Enneagram as a pragmatic tool, adding his own insights and discoveries, and with Russ Hudson developed the Riso-Hudson Enneagram Type Indicator (RHETI), an empirically validated questionnaire for assessing one's dominant personality type. We highly encourage you to take the online version of the RHETI for a nominal fee at www.enneagraminstitute.com. The questionnaire involves responding to 144 pairs of forced-choice statements that will take about 40 minutes to complete and will offer a unique and comprehensive portrait of your dominant personality type, including a full-spectrum report indicating the relative strengths and weaknesses of the nine types within your overall personality, and personal growth recommendations for your specific dominant type.

As this chapter provides only a brief introduction to the Enneagram, we encourage you to consult the Enneagram Institute at the above-referenced Web site for a more detailed discussion of the history of the Enneagram and expanded descriptions of the nine personality types. Riso and Hudson's seminal works *The Wisdom of the Enneagram: The Complete Guide to the Psychological and Spiritual Growth for the Nine Personality Types* (1999) and *Discovering Your Personality Type* (2003; includes a self-administered paper-and-pencil version of the RHETI) are must-have texts if you intend to use the Enneagram to develop and implement treatment plans for your clients seeking permanent habit control.

Although understanding our dominant personality type can be extremely enlightening and beneficial for enhancing the quality of our lives, it is important to understand that everyone contains within themselves aspects of the other eight personality types. As intended with the Enneagram, we don't want to get trapped in a type-casting mentality where gaining a better understanding of ourselves ends with "cookbook interpretations." Riso and Hudson (2003) remind us: "When we speak of our type it is useful to think of it as our *dominant* type—our default setting and motivational core. This is an extremely valuable thing to know, and it can greatly facilitate our growth by being aware of what is most centrally driving our ego agendas" (p. 9).

Ultimately, the power of the Enneagram comes from discovering our dominant personality type and "courageously observing ourselves as we really are, no matter what we find" (Riso & Hudson, 2003, p. 10). Living a life that is *present* focused, abiding in the here-and-now, while objectively observing our personalities in action, provides the key for transformation. With this knowledge, individuals desiring to change unwanted habits can become more mindful of the internal and external drives and perceptions that bind them to their behaviors. Likewise, the act of bringing awareness to the moment allows the higher essential qualities of the self to be mobilized, which in turn fosters and promotes emotional and spiritual growth.

The RHETI Sampler Personality Test, which can be taken online at no cost at The Enneagram Institute Web site can be scored instantly and offers an opportunity for initial insight into one's personality type. The Sampler, like the complete RHETI, is a forced-choice test that requires you to circle the letter corresponding to one statement in each pair of statements that describes you best and applies to you through *most of your life.*

The Sampler, unlike the full RHETI, has NOT been scientifically validated. However, in most cases your highest score will likely reflect your basic type or, at the very least, be among the top three scores. If nothing else, it can help you and your clients begin a journey of self-discovery!

How The System Works

At first glance, the Enneagram's structure appears complicated. However, it is surprisingly simple. As you can see (Figure 3.1), the nine points, each representing a core or dominant personality trait, are con-

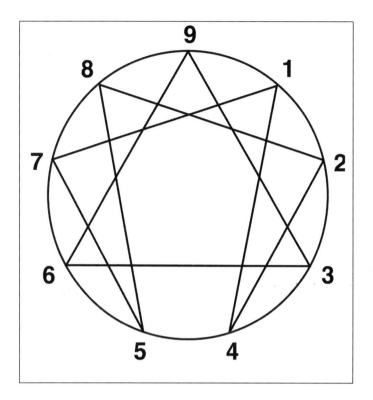

Figure 3.1 The Enneagram. Copyright 2009. The Enneagram Institute. All rights reserved. Used with permission.

nected with each other by inner lines. Note that points Three, Six, and Nine form an equilateral triangle. The remaining six points are connected as follows: One connects with Four, Four with Two, Two with Eight, Eight with Five, Five with Seven, and Seven with One. The meanings of the lines and their interrelationship will be reviewed shortly.

According to Riso and Hudson (1999, 2003), we all emerge from childhood with one of the nine types dominating our personality. In fact, most of the major Enneagram authors agree that we are born with a dominant type. Consequently, this inborn core personality structure largely determines how we learn to adapt to and perceive our environment, which in turn influences the development of core defense mechanisms. It should be noted, though, that there is an understanding that we possess "energy" of all nine types within us.

As we mentioned previously, no single type is preferable or better than the other. For this reason, a value-neutral numbering system is employed to designate each personality type. Ultimately, the health of our personality type can be measured by our self-awareness, our mindfulness, and capacity to be present in the here-and-now. Unlike the more familiar psychiatric nomenclature that relies on labels to describe personality types, the nominal system of the Enneagram offers an unbiased, shorthand way of objectively describing an individual without assuming or implying pathology.

In general, it is understood that people do not change from one personality type to another—again, no one type is healthier or better than another—though it is certainly possible to change and develop over time as we grow emotionally and develop healthier coping skills. In essence, each type has varying degrees of health that Riso and Hudson refer to as Levels of Development (2003). Each type has unique capacities and abilities as well as limitations and impediments to personal growth. Ultimately, the value of the Enneagram is in understanding the self as thoroughly as possible and striving to be *the best self* through awareness and mindfulness and not imitating preferred assets of another personality type.

Some personality typology theories and systems rely on gender and age-based normative references. Although it may be tempting to assign gender characteristics to the Enneagram, it is a system that is universal, applying equally to males and females, without any type being identified as inherently masculine or feminine.

Identifying Your Basic Personality Type

At this time, if you have not already done so, we encourage you to take time to take the RHETI (www.enneagraminstitute.com) as insight into your basic personality type will offer a more pragmatic, "hands-on" understanding of the Enneagram.

If you pass on the invitation to take the RHETI, as you consider what you understand about your personality, which of the following nine "roles" in Figure 3.2 describes you best *most of the time*? It is important to recognize and consider your dominant personality role

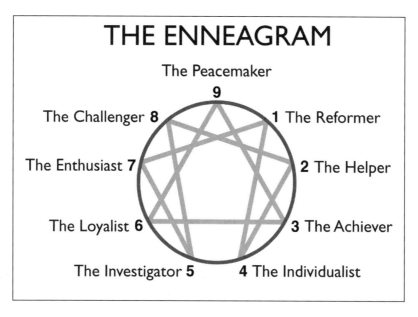

THE ENNEAGRAM

The Peacemaker

9

The Challenger **8** — **1** The Reformer

The Enthusiast **7** — **2** The Helper

The Loyalist **6** — **3** The Achiever

The Investigator **5** — **4** The Individualist

Figure 3.2 The Enneagram with Riso-Hudson type names. Copyright 2009. The Enneagram Institute. All rights reserved. Used with permission.

throughout your entire life, and not how and where you may be presently—or, more importantly, not how or where you *want* to be.

Which of the following sets of personality traits best characterizes your personality?

- Type One, **The Reformer**—principled, purposeful, self-controlled, perfectionistic
- Type Two, **The Helper**—generous, demonstrative, people-pleasing, possessive
- Type Three, **The Achiever**—adaptable, excelling, driven, image conscious
- Type Four, **The Individualist**—expressive, dramatic, self-absorbed, temperamental
- Type Five, **The Investigator**—perceptive, innovative, secretive, isolated
- Type Six, **The Loyalist**—engaging, responsible, anxious, suspicious

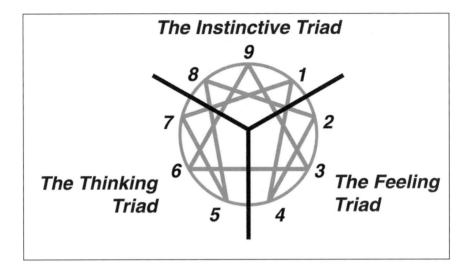

Figure 3.3 The triads of the Enneagram. Copyright 2009. The Enneagram Institute. All rights reserved. Used with permission.

- Type Seven, **The Enthusiast**—spontaneous, versatile, distractible, scattered
- Type Eight, **The Challenger**—self-confident, decisive, willful, confrontational
- Type Nine, **The Peacemaker**—receptive, reassuring, accommodating, complacent

The TRIADS

The Enneagram is a three-by-three grid of nine personality types separated into three triads: the **Instinctive Triad**, the **Feeling Triad**, and the **Thinking Triad**. Each Triad consists of three personality types that share the assets and liabilities of that Triad. For instance, Type Three has unique strengths and challenges involving its feelings and for this reason is found within the Feeling Triad along with Type Two and Type Four. Similarly, Type Six's assets and liabilities involve its relationship to more instinctual drives and, along with types Five and Seven, is in the Thinking Triad.

Each type can be described as having a cluster of issues or shared emotional experiences that characterize a Triad (Figure 3.3). In essence, each Triad has issues that develop from a largely unconscious emotional response arising from the loss of contact with the core self. For instance, *anger* or *rage* characterize the underlying emotion of the Instinctive Triad; *shame* is the primary emotion in the Feeling Triad; and *anxiety* fuels the types within the Thinking Triad.

The personality types within the Instinctive Triad (Eight, Nine, and One), or what Brian refers to as "the belly-based center types," want to impact, affect, and control their environments without being impacted or controlled in return. In each of these types, there are three unique ways of dealing with the issue of control. One way is by being assertive, another by withdrawing, and a third by earning the privilege to control.

More specifically, **Eights** deal with ensuring autonomy and respect by engaging in overtly aggressive behaviors—raising their voices, shouting, moving forcefully and in a threatening manner. In contrast, **Nines** withdraw for autonomy and deny their anger and instinctual energies. Nines essentially retreat from their darker side by focusing on idealizations of their relationships and their universe. **Ones** on the other hand, earn autonomy. They "do the right thing" so no one can tell them what to do. Ones respond to their inner critic (i.e., superego) in ways that influence perfectionist traits that are employed to suppress their hostile and angry feelings.

The Wings

There is general agreement among those well versed in the Enneagram that no individual can be defined by a single dominant type. Everyone is a unique mixture of a dominant personality type and usually *one* of the types adjacent to it. The two types adjacent to each identified dominant type are referred to as wings. For instance Threes have either a Two-wing or a Four-wing, Fours have either a Three-wing or a Five-wing, and so forth. Ultimately, the wings help individualize the nine general types. Though some purport that everyone in essence has two wings, general consensus is that one wing is dominant and serves as the identified subtype to the dominant type. That being said, it is possible that an individual may not have a dominant wing and that, indeed, both wings would be relevant, though this is less common.

The dominant type characterizes the overall personality and the wing complements it, adding important and sometimes contradictory elements to the total personality. The wing can be considered the "second side" of the personality, which permits a more robust understanding of an individual. Take for instance someone who has a dominant personality type Three. As noted above, this person will likely have either a Two-wing or a Four-wing that further defines and characterizes the personality.

More specific discussion, offering an in-depth understanding of the wings, is beyond the scope of this chapter. You are encouraged to consult Riso and Hudson's *The Wisdom of the Enneagram* (1999). In this seminal work, the authors painstakingly review the nine personality types and the two wings affiliated with each type. They identify more specific personality characteristics for each personality type, their wings, behavioral descriptions of the levels of development for each type, and pragmatic recommendations for integrating each personality type.

Levels of Development

Arguably the most unique contribution to the Enneagram of Personality Types by Riso and subsequently developed by Hudson is the Levels of Development. The Levels of Development, as described by Riso and Hudson in *Discovering Your Personality Type* (2003), "account for differences between people of the same type as well as how people change both for better or worse" (p. 76).

The Levels of Development provide a framework for understanding how the traits of each type are interrelated and how these traits can possibly deteriorate into dysfunctional traits or grow and prosper, manifesting a healthier, highly effective functioning personality. By including the levels, the Enneagram, once a flat, horizontal set of nine discrete categories, becomes a multidimensional system (Figure 3.4).

With the inclusion of the Levels, the Enneagram becomes more reflective of the changing nature of personality patterns. Just as our moods, behaviors, beliefs, attitudes, and life philosophies change— sometimes we think more clearly and live a grounded, emotionally available life; at other times we may stew in anxiety or engage in rigid, resistant, reactive, and emotionally volatile behaviors—so too does our level of development within our dominant personality type.

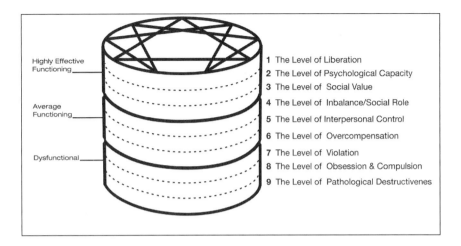

Highly Effective Functioning

Average Functioning

Dysfunctional

1 The Level of Liberation
2 The Level of Psychological Capacity
3 The Level of Social Value
4 The Level of Inbalance/Social Role
5 The Level of Interpersonal Control
6 The Level of Overcompensation
7 The Level of Violation
8 The Level of Obsession & Compulsion
9 The Level of Pathological Destructivenes

Figure 3.4 The continuum of the levels of development. Copyright 2009. The Enneagram Institute. All rights reserved. Used with permission.

To more fully understand ourselves and others, as well as more effectively relate with one another, it is necessary to accurately perceive where a person lies along the continuum of levels within a personality type. Individuals with the same dominant type may look very different from each other if one person exists in a healthy range of functioning while the other is living an average or unhealthy existence. When working with individuals to promote habit change, it is crucial to gain an understanding of their Level of Development, as therapeutic interventions will be designed with one primary goal in mind: moving the person up the continuum to healthier levels of development. In so doing, we help liberate them from the habit(s) that reflect lower levels of functioning and unhealthy levels of development.

At each level, significant psychological shifts occur. Riso and Hudson have labeled each level to connote the nature of the shift. For example, at Level Five, the Level of Interpersonal Control, an individual, no matter what their dominant personality type, is trying to manipulate the self and others to get his or her needs met, which of course generates interpersonal conflict. Level Five is ego driven. Essentially, the person is fully identified with the ego and will increasingly defend and inflate the ego to feel safe and keep his or her identity preserved. If ample stress persists or increases, the person may deteriorate to a Level Six, the Level of Overcompensation, where behaviors regress and become aggressive and intrusive. At this level, the ego is fragile and will engage in increasingly dysfunctional behaviors to have its needs met, regardless of the impact it may have on others.

The more we move down the Levels of Development, the more we identify with our ego and its negative and destructive behavioral patterns. At lower levels, our personality becomes more defensive, reactive, less conscious of our current existence, and ultimately destructive, not only toward ourselves, but toward others. In contrast, as we become more present and attuned to ourselves and our environment, the less defensive and restricted we become and the more detached we become from the disabling aspects of our personality.

Directions of Integration (Security) and Disintegration (Stress)

Just as the Levels of Development are fluid, and change over time, the inner lines of the Enneagram connect the different types in a sequence that identifies what each type will do under certain circumstances. Note in Figure 3.2 how each type has two lines projecting from it toward another type. One line connects with another type in a way that represents how a person is expected to behave when he or she feels more secure and in control of a situation (Direction of Integration). The second line represents the Direction of Disintegration and represents how a person is likely to act out under increased or prolonged stress that seems overwhelming and unmanageable.

The Direction of Integration (see Figure 3.5) for each type is indicated by the sequence of numbers 1-7-5-8-2-4-1 and 9-3-6-9: an integrating One goes to Seven; an integrating Seven goes to Five; an integrating Five goes to Eight; an integrating Eight goes to Two; an integrating Two goes to Four; and an integrating Four goes to One. On the equilateral triangle portion of the Enneagram, an integrating Nine goes to Three; an integrating Three goes to Six; and an integrating Six goes to Nine.

The Direction of Disintegration for each type is indicated as the *reverse* of the sequences for Integration and is as follows: 1-4-2-8-5-7-1 and 9-6-3-9. Consequently, when under stress, an average-to-unhealthy One will behave like an average-to-unhealthy Four; an average-to-

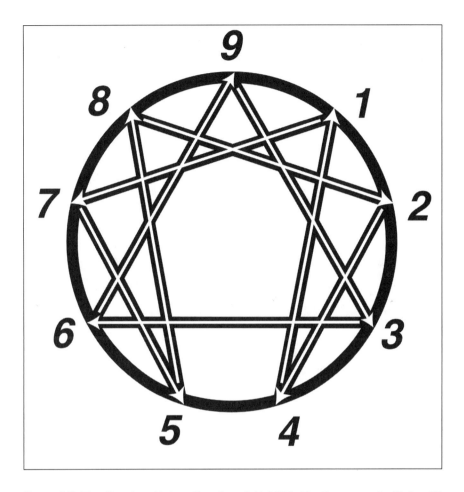

Figure 3.5 The direction of integration. Copyright 2009. The Enneagram Institute. All rights reserved. Used with permission.

unhealthy Four will respond to stress much like an average-to-unhealthy Two, and so forth. Figure 3.6 represents The Direction of Disintegration for all nine types.

THE ENNEAGRAM AND HABIT CONTROL

As this is a text about habit control, we will focus efforts and attention on understanding how habit-related behaviors, attitudes, and treatment

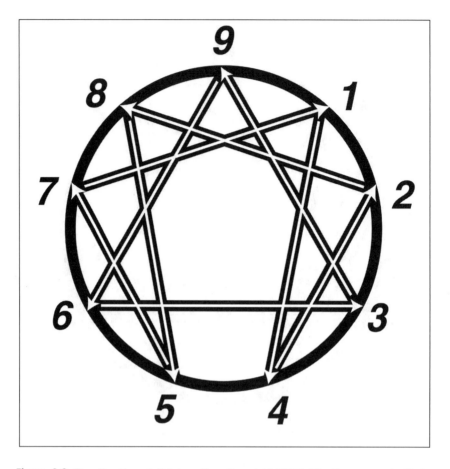

Figure 3.6 The direction of disintegration. Copyright 2009. The Enneagram Institute. All rights reserved. Used with permission.

of unwanted habits are influenced by the core Enneagram Personality Type of the client. As it will no doubt become clear to you, the Enneagram—and more specifically the RHETI—is a clinical and therapeutic tool that can offer profound insight for anyone desiring change in their life, whether that change involves an unwanted habit, or improved relations with others, or opportunities for emotional and spiritual growth.

It is also important to recognize and appreciate (though we do not dedicate much time to it in this chapter) how our own Enneagram type influences our relationships with our clients, including the course and possible outcome of our therapeutic endeavors. If, for example, your dominant personality type is Eight, the flow of the therapy session is likely to be very direct, authoritative, maybe even confrontational. Type Eight therapists are also likely to establish and maintain a set of expectations from their clients that when unmet generate a sense of frustration for the therapist. This, of course, we know and understand as countertransference. If you are not cognizant of these countertransference experiences, particularly those that are more prone to occur when treating certain personality types (e.g., Type Two), therapy is likely to be counterproductive or progress impeded at the very least.

We now turn our attention to the characteristics of each of the nine Enneagram personality types. We will conclude the overview of each personality type with information that is more individualized and relevant to habit-control treatment. Again, although this chapter offers a brief overview of the Enneagram of Personality Types, we encourage you to supplement this information by perusing other and more comprehensive Enneagram references mentioned throughout this chapter.

The Instinctive Triad

The Instinctive, or Gut, Triad operates on an underlying emotion of anger or rage. Eights act out their anger, typically in some physically aggressive or overpowering manner; Nines deny their anger and are essentially out of touch with their emotions; and Ones attempt to control their anger through repression and control of their environment (see Figure 3.7).

Type Eight

Type Eight, The Challenger, is also known as the powerful-dominating type. Though other types have traits and characteristics that involve elements of power and dominance, the essence of Type Eight is the exertion of power and dominance over others. Eights can be strong, assertive, action oriented, competitive, and insistent. They encounter conflict with others because they can be willful, defiant, and confrontational. But it is their honorable nature, generous attitude, and inspiring character that can make them beneficial to others when they operate at fully functioning, healthier levels.

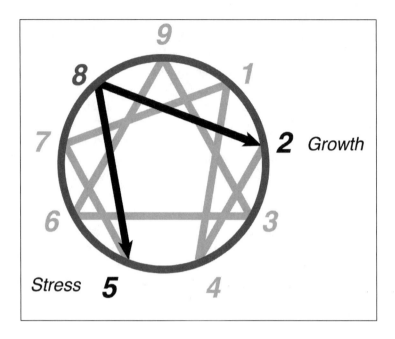

Figure 3.7 Type Eight: The Challenger. Copyright 2009. The Enneagram Institute. All rights reserved. Used with permission.

As you will see, each personality type has an elementary fear that is imbedded within the unconscious mind and involves a basic fear of a *loss of being*. It is what some have called the "primal catastrophe." And each type will interpret that loss of being, or loss of oneness, in different ways.

For Eights, the fear involves being harmed, violated, or betrayed. At its core, it is the fear of being controlled or dominated by others. Eights perceive the self as having been violated or taken advantage of, consequently Eights remain motivated to be strong and self-reliant, to control and protect the self, to dominate and prevail over others when necessary. Eights operate under the assumption that the best defense is a first-strike, preemptive offense.

For each type we consider what it is that that type is "in search of." Eights are in search of impact, of being real and seeking intensity that comes from giving and taking on challenges. Eights are action-oriented personalities who externalize and engage in sensory-motor processing.

Eights tend to have a disproportionate impact on the world, both for good or for bad, depending on the health of the personality, and can be evidenced in assertive humans such as Martin Luther King, Jr., Theodore Roosevelt, and Donald Trump. They are generally strong, assertive, resourceful, independent, determined, shrewd, straight talking, and insistent. At their best, they are honorable, heroic, empowering, generous, decisive, and inspiring. But when distressed or in conflict, Eights may regress to being blunt, willful, domineering, forceful, defiant, confrontational, bad tempered, cynical, and vengeful.

Type Eight exemplifies the desire to be independent, maintain a "can-do, get-it-done" attitude. They are determined to be self-reliant and free to pursue their own destiny, no matter what. They tend to be natural leaders who are gifted at seeing the possibilities in others and tapping into others' strengths and abilities. Honor is very important to Eights, as their word is their bond. They can be very honorable, but usually on their own terms and not when dictated to by others.

Healthy Eights are visionaries who often engage in money-making projects or business ventures and can thrive on taking risks. When moving toward a direction of security, healthy Eights may look like average Twos and seek support from others, relying and depending on confidants for assistance that otherwise may be perceived as a sign of weakness by an unhealthy Eight. As they recognize how their defensiveness limits their development, Eights can become more emotionally expressive and generous, like high functioning Twos.

At their worst, Eights can be controlling, demanding and willful and can engage in bullying behaviors when it suits them to do so. When under significant distress they may decompensate and become isolative, looking like Average Fives as they become strangely quiet and secretive while privately managing their problems.

Eights grow by recognizing that not everything is a battle or fight to win. They realize that life is not about "survival of the fittest" and that strength actually involves a sense of vulnerability and openness to others. Eights grow by recognizing that more can be accomplished through employing a cooperative spirit than by struggling against others and doing all things independently.

Habit Control Work With Eights. Eights are intense, competitive individuals who live life large and hard. Eights live an existence where "more is better." For Eights, if one drink is good, two drinks are better, four drinks would be best. This type of analogy can be applied to many behaviors, including overeating, alcohol overconsumption, reckless driving, and overindulgence. Through their behaviors Eights can be "larger than life," taking up and using more space and energy than is really necessary. Anything that seems middle-of-the-road is boring for Eights.

It is also true that Eights do not like restraints imposed on them, therefore they are prone to ignore medical concerns out of fear that they may be controlled by a physician or other health care provider whom they believe will *impose* unwelcomed advice. This advice will be particularly troublesome for Eights if it involves some kind of restriction or imposition on their lifestyle that slows them down or interferes with their goals and objectives in life.

Eights tend to be very self-reliant and refuse to engage in behaviors that can be characterized as dependent or passive. With this in mind, we find it is particularly helpful to put Eights into action by assigning them tasks that potentiate the competitive nature of their very being. For instance, with Eights who are motivated to becoming permanent nonsmokers, we challenge them to put their cigarettes in inconvenient places (e.g., the top shelf of the kitchen cabinet, behind some dishes, the trunk of their car while driving). This challenge allows them to pause for a moment to decide if they want to go through the trouble to get a cigarette when perhaps they could actually do without one. David has also found it helpful to encourage Eights to smoke with their opposite hand. Though a simple intervention that could be readily declined, it will make smoking a bit more awkward, at times to the extent that the person would rather not smoke.

It is generally common knowledge and clearly established that Type A personalities (i.e.,Eights) are more prone to heart attacks because of their persistent drive, ambition, and overly competitive nature. Interestingly, Type A's who survive heart attacks are less likely to have another one because they become motivated and driven to do all that is necessary to minimize the risk of having a second heart attack. This finding was first identified in the Western Collaborative Group Study (Rosenman et al., 1975), which followed 3,154 healthy men between ages 39 and 59 for 8 years. The primary finding was that the men who displayed Type A behavior at the beginning of the study were twice as likely to develop coronary heart disease as the men with Type B (relaxed, non-competitive) behavior patterns. When the investigators analyzed the data for the younger men, they discovered that this risk was six times as high for Type A personalities. Interestingly, a subsequent study conducted by Ragland and Brand (1988) reported a 22-year follow-up of the men in the Western Collaborative Group Study. They found that individuals with Type B personality were likely to have a second heart attack earlier than Type A individuals.

It is essential to be direct and active with Eights, to stand up to them, and be assertive—though not necessarily confrontational—with them. Eights respect people who are direct, honest, and say what they mean and mean what they say.

In due time, Eights will surrender the sense of needing to be in control if they have confidence in you as a therapist. If, however, you are not direct, active, and assertive, it will be difficult for them to confide in and trust you. In general, enhancing compassion, restraint, and vulnerability in therapy will facilitate growth for Eights, for they tend to be interpersonally protected and defended.

For Eights, grief work is critical, as they tend to maintain a "hard shell" to protect themselves from feeling much of anything. They may have developed a habit that in some ways serves to protect them, therefore it is helpful for Eights to process their feelings in ways that allows them to gain distance from their unwanted habit. Eights who are smokers, for instance, may be seen as angry and bitter and turn to their cigarettes to keep people away through toxic smoke they exhale.

Eights should also be encouraged to retreat to more peaceful experiences, perhaps through meditation so they can quiet their minds and revitalize their senses. Eights can respond very well to hypnosis as they tend to challenge themselves to go deeper into trance, desiring the benefits of hypnosis by getting into the best possible trance state.

Eights who desire healthier bodies will respond well to coaching if they are not acquainted with exercise, particularly anaerobic weight training. Providing Eights with references on the most effective weight training strategies (e.g., pyramid training, overload principle, prioritization of muscle groups, etc.) will enhance their individual abilities to obtain the ideal body they seek. Because Eights respond well to authority figures who not only talk-the-talk, but walk-the-walk, pairing them with a fitness "coach" or instructor can be very beneficial and rewarding.

Remember, above all else, even though Eights can and do throw their weight around, they respond best to direct, honest, straightforward feedback and information. If you tend to be a more timid or cerebral therapist, who likes to analyze and solve problems much like a Type

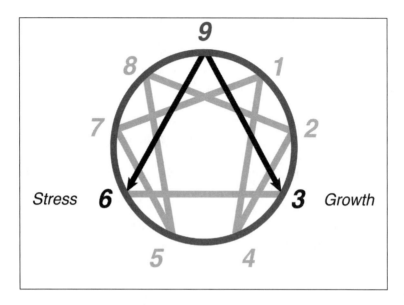

Figure 3.8 Type Nine: The Peacemaker. Copyright 2009. The Enneagram Institute. All rights reserved. Used with permission.

Five, you will want to learn a thing or two from Eights so that you can become more directive and assertive in your therapy with them.

Type Nine

Sometimes called the mediator or the pleasant self-effacing type, Nines are receptive, reassuring, complacent, and resigned. They are seen as steady, easygoing, agreeable, and sensual; however, they find themselves in conflict with others because they can be emotionally unavailable, inattentive, and stubborn. When functioning well, Nines are appreciated for their capacity to be self-aware, imaginative, passionate, and proactive.

The basic fear for Nines is being "cut off from the mother ship," so to speak. It is about losing the peace, about disconnection and fragmentation. Because Nines are afraid of disconnection, fragmentation, and losing their peace, they strongly desire union, harmony, and personal peace and remain motivated to avoid conflicts and ignore anything that would be upsetting.

Nines are persistent optimists, typically seeking the best in others, while hoping for the best for themselves. They seek the end of the rainbow, wanting every story to have a happy ending, only to be frequently disappointed.

Average Nines prefer a simple and uncomplicated existence. Average Nines frequently "bite their tongue" reserving their own opinions and reactions; however, they can be quite assertive on behalf of others and will work very diligently if it is of benefit to other people.

Nines desire peace, wholeness, and harmony in the world and as a result they are generally easygoing, emotionally stable, and patient with themselves and others. Regardless of the circumstances or dysfunction of the environment surrounding them, Nines strive to bring everything and everyone back to a harmonious unity.

In their relationships with others, Nines fear conflict and will internalize tension and uncomfortable feelings before expressing their true feelings. When it seems too much for them, however, Nines can become very volatile and "blow up" seemingly out of the blue. Others may be surprised by their reaction and behavior, as it is likely to seem out of character.

At their best, Nines assert themselves more freely and experience even greater peace and contentment, as it comes from a very real place that is devoid of anxiety associated with rejection or disappointment. Healthy Nines begin to understand that their very existence makes them valuable, as they begin to perceive the positive impact that they have upon their environment. As such, like healthy Threes, they begin to invest time and energy in themselves and learn to take pleasure in their own value and goodness.

When seeking security during times of distress and uncertainty, Nines avoid conflict by detaching emotionally and engaging in more isolative behavior. At such times, their behavior appears more reminiscent of an average-to-unhealthy Six. They become worried, testy, and interpersonally defensive. They project blame for their difficulties onto others and, like an unhealthy six, will complain to anyone who will listen.

Nines grow when they finally understand that avoiding the problems and conflicts in life simply generates greater unhappiness and dysfunction in their relationships. Ultimately, they learn that their avoidance of conflict is the very thing that generates conflict with others. When they begin to apply assertiveness effectively, recognizing that there really is a difference between assertion and aggression, they will be in a better position to promote the sense of peace and harmony they are seeking with others.

Habit Control Work With Nines. By nature, Nines are avoidant. They may avoid conflict, confrontation, and just about any kind of pressure to initiate change. Their avoidance manifests itself through "narcotizing," zoning out, daydreaming, and dissociating. Although this avoidance in and of itself makes for therapeutic obstacles, as we discuss below, Nines, because they are good at "zoning out," can be excellent hypnotherapy candidates. Essentially, they move through life in a trance, albeit a negative and self-destructive one.

Though any of the types may dissociate in their own way, Nines are prone to dissociation through daydreaming. They have a particular propensity for using and abusing sweets, alcohol, and other substances that provide a temporary, yet pleasant "buzz" to help get them through the day and distance them from any sense of conflict.

As we discussed previously, it is also important for Nines to suppress their anger. Consequently, they tend to stuff themselves with food, cigarettes, and alcohol. They tend to be unaware of what they are doing, consequently their behaviors seem to occur on more of a subconscious level. For instance, they may check the refrigerator or pantry for a snack without much forethought or consideration of the fact that they may be doing so, even when they are not hungry.

Nines also tend to be "other-oriented" or at least not self-oriented. They are great cheerleaders for others, but when it comes to accessing a sense of internal motivation and drive, unlike Eights, Nines fall short when it comes to taking care of themselves and putting themselves first. They tend to behave in ways that exhibit an unending supply of patience; however, closer scrutiny of an unhealthy Nine reveals chronic procrastination when it comes to doing something for themselves.

Nines are, however, capable of seeing the big picture, and as therapists we can get them to buy into this bigger picture, by using their patience to stick with the established plan. In this way, hypnotherapy can be helpful when it incorporates projection into the future. Using trance work that involves elements of having an individual imagine the body they want capitalizes upon Nines' ability to consider the big picture. It is also helpful, as we discuss in our chapter on hypnosis, to include multisensory modalities. For instance, we can employ visualization by having a client imagine how he will *look*; tactile imagery by having him imagine how he will *feel* or how his clothes fit; and auditory imagery by helping him imagine what he will *hear* other people say to him as he walks around in his ideal body. We are essentially helping him set the stage for the body he wants, much like athletes visualize the performance and outcome they desire.

Nines tend to be very receptive and accepting of suggestions and advice. When working with Nines, it is important to present a peaceful, agreeable, unifying perspective that helps them understand and realize how managing their unwanted habits is going to provide them with a greater sense of comfort, peace, and security.

Because Nines are known as Peacemakers, it is important in our therapy with them to help them learn the value and power of the word *no*. Nines tend to take on more than they can handle, thereby generating unnecessary stress that only enhances the likelihood of engaging in unhealthy habits like smoking or overeating. It is also beneficial for Nines to appreciate that people would rather they be direct and express their opinion or preference rather than resist others through passive-aggressive behaviors after making a commitment that can't be kept or, if kept, is done so with resentment.

Type One

A Type One person is sometimes called the perfectionist or the judge, the rational idealistic type—principled, purposeful, self-controlled, and critical. Remember, Ones, like Eights and Nines, are "gut" type personalities who respond on the level of instinctive feelings. For Ones, the elementary fear is the fear of being wrong, corrupt, or defective, so the motivating desire is to be "good," to do "right," and ultimately to avoid criticism of any kind. Conflict ensues when their character becomes opinionated, impatient, irritable, and sarcastic. But when Ones are functioning well, they are appreciated for their tolerance, acceptance, and a willingness to delay reinforcement for a higher good.

By maintaining a belief that they can be perfect, Ones work diligently to do what they believe is the good and right thing to do, so that they can avoid being criticized. Frequently comparing themselves with some ideal of perfection generates a sense of frustration and disappointment for Ones—with themselves and with others for not being equally punc-

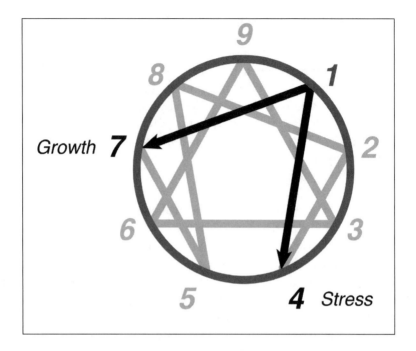

Figure 3.9 Type One: The Reformer. Copyright 2009. The Enneagram Institute. All rights reserved. Used with permission.

tual, efficient, and particular about details. Another source of frustration for Ones is the assumption that they are responsible for making sure everything is perfect, that the *i*'s are dotted and the *t*'s are crossed, while everyone else just doesn't seem to care that much. In their minds, they have to be the adults and take responsibility, as it is apparent to them that no one else will. Over time, Ones become resentful, frustrated, and disappointed as they fail to live up to their own exacting standards.

Ones are very thorough and generally well organized. Some Ones maintain an extraordinary concern for neatness, living the dictum that "everything has its place and every place has its thing." Ones are not too difficult to spot, as they have everything organized at the office, where all pencils are sharpened and file folders are labeled and filed alphabetically, and at home, where socks and underwear are neatly folded and stacked, if not occasionally rotated to ensure even wear and tear. Felix Unger, the eternal neatnick, from Neil Simon's play *The Odd*

Couple, immediately comes to mind as an appropriate characterization of a Type One.

When Ones become less strict with themselves and lower their perfectionist expectations, they enjoy a greater sense of freedom and spontaneity, much like healthy Sevens. Their direction of integration is more like that of a healthy Seven who lives the maxim, "Whatever is worth doing is worth doing badly." They lighten up on the "must" and "should" demands of the superego and instead recognize what they want.

Unhealthy Ones can be impatient, irritable, angry, rigid, sarcastic, and judgmental. Under stress, they feel misunderstood and unappreciated by their peers and often withdraw from others to sort out their feelings, much like average-to-unhealthy Fours. When feeling bitter and depressed, Ones often turn to self-indulgent behavior in an attempt to relieve their uncomfortable feelings. For example, a One who is a compulsive health nut who exercises regularly and maintains a strict low-fat, low-carb diet, might start indulging in milk shakes or candy bars. Typically, this behavior produces guilt, leaving the One more depressed and self-critical, and possibly initiating a snowball effect of self-destructive behavior.

Ones grow by appreciating that others take things seriously too, but that their own approach has been a bit over-the-top and extreme. Ones also grow by living more spontaneously and engaging in recreational activities that promote a sense of freedom from their expectations of perfection. Once they fully understand and accept reality with all its imperfections and contradictions, they can begin to grow by simply *accepting what is.*

Habit Control Work With Ones.   Habit issues with Ones are generally related to a strict superego that may fuel unrealistic expectations and perfectionism. They are people who operate on instinct and passion with convictions and judgments that control and direct themselves and their actions. Though the superego plays an important role for each type, Ones can lay claim to the lion's share of owning a strong, rigid, strict superego that sits upon their shoulder, constantly telling them, "Do this!...Don't do that!...That's bad!...That's good!...That's right!... That's wrong!"

With strong superegos comes resistance to changing behaviors, even if those behaviors are habits that are unhealthy and unwanted.

By the same token, habits for Ones could be reactions against the strict superego. Like a willful child acting out against a disciplinarian parent, Ones are known for their perfectionism and the self-imposed pressures that require valves that can be opened once in a while to let off the building pressure. Drinking, gambling, or overeating, for instance, become safety valves or escape hatches for that kind of pressure.

Under severe and pathological conditions, the rigid superego of Ones can develop eating disorders through their attempts to overcontrol that which is ultimately in their control, such as what they do or do not choose to put in their mouths (e.g., food). Compulsive exercise, severe dietary restrictions, or—quite the contrary—binging and purging behaviors are examples of pathological Ones losing control through their attempts to overcontrol. If in your work as a therapist you tend to treat individuals with eating disorders, you will likely encounter your fair share of Ones and need to help them settle their superegos.

Ones are also known for maintaining an *all-or-nothing* perspective on life. They believe that they must be scrupulously self-controlled at all times, but if they are not able to do this, their perspective may be that nothing can be controlled. Failing to live up to their own standards generates intense guilt, which may then result in the development and maintenance of unwanted habits.

On a subconscious level, Ones are what Freud referred to as "anal retentive." They may have issues with their bodies and bodily functions and may have been taught that they and their biological needs are *messy* and something to be ashamed of. They may respond to these messages by being ultraclean, ultracareful, ultrascrupulous, and hypervigilent about themselves and their bodies. Closer scrutiny may reveal rebellion against the superego and in fact, situations like this, much to the chagrin or perhaps entertainment of the general public, make for national headlines, such as when the dirty laundry aired by the news media exposes the conservative, "pro-family" politician who engaged in secret homosexual activities in a public restroom, or the priest whose homily denounces child abuse hours before doing unthinkable things to an innocent child, or the political commentator who condemns substance abusers when he himself is addicted to prescriptive medication. Of course, these are extreme examples of rebellion against the superego, but they readily make the point.

On a less pathological level, we may find the industrious and proper workaholic office manager taking a secret weekend to Las Vegas or the straightlaced housewife who lets her hair down on a weekend night as she bar–hops, looking for a bit more excitement in her life.

It is important to realize that although this discipline, this rigid sense of responsibility can generate unwanted pressure and unhealthy habits, it can also be very helpful in therapy if used to the person's advantage. Ones maintain a sense of commitment and accountability that if they decide to make changes in their lives, including healthy diet and exercise, they are very capable of staying focused and determined to accomplish their goals. Additionally, Ones are very competent organizers and can make good use of time and energy, a trait that can be used therapeutically.

Ones are adept at following through with procedures, so in therapy it can be very beneficial to provide them with structured, clearly specified, concrete, and objective assignments. Having them monitor progress, take notes, or keep a journal can be helpful, though one must be careful of the "all-or-nothing" attitude that could create havoc for Ones if they do not believe they are progressing. It is therefore important to be as certain as possible that the superego is tamed to the extent that the person understands there are *shades of gray* in life and that not everything *must* be perfect.

Ones also tend to want to get down to business and get things done, consequently small talk about the weather or newsworthy events is unnecessary and generally perceived by them as a waste of their time. They are likely to take notes in therapy or bring notes with them for their therapy session. Maintaining a sense of organization and ensuring that they work through that "things to discuss" list in therapy is important for Ones. As therapists, we should encourage this and not respond by telling them that notes are distracting or unnecessary.

Because Ones tend to maintain a level of hypervigalence, they are good at scanning their environments and evaluating circumstances in their lives. Unfortunately, less healthy Ones tend to scan for the negatives, being ever mindful of what they are doing wrong or what isn't going right in their life. As therapists, we can help them "scan" for what is positive or for indications of personal growth and progress.

Rigid superegos resist fun and relaxation, sending the message of what the person "should" be doing rather than what they "want" to do. If there is a want or desire, the superego of Ones tells them it is wrong. In therapy with Ones we strive to relax the superego, helping the person be less critical of self and others, working through a process of forgiveness when necessary. Ones tend to *resent* others for what they did or did not do for them and *regret* what they did or did not do that now leads to disappointment. To heal these feelings of resentment and regret, forgiveness must be instituted and become a critical component of therapy. When true forgiveness occurs, Ones (and others) can be less critical of themselves and others. They are able to let go of the baggage they carry that likely reinforces the unwanted and unhealthy habit they want to change.

As David tells his clients struggling with their superego, "Get Judge Judy out of your head, and rent some space to the likes of Gandhi, Jesus, Nelson Mandela, or others who exemplified the healing nature of forgiveness."

Therapists who are themselves Ones run the risk of countertransference issues that could impede therapy. If you have a strong or rigid sense of right and wrong, good and bad, it may be difficult to be objective with clients who struggle with their own superegos. It is therefore critical to be aware of your own beliefs and perceptions and to maintain a professional distance and sense of objectivity that doesn't reinforce the very thought processes and behaviors that generate conflict for your client. Learning to live a more spontaneous life, accepting things as they are at times, and being more carefree in your own personal experience can be helpful for minimizing the countertransference issues that can arise when helping Ones overcome unwanted habits.

The Feeling Triad

Although the types comprising the Instinctive/Gut Triad share an underlying emotion of anger, the Feeling/Heart Triad, comprising Personality Types Two, Three, and Four, shares an underlying emotion of shame. Twos compensate for their underlying shame by getting others to approve and like them, Threes work diligently at denying their shame through overcompensation and attempts to achieve success, and Fours avoid their shame by focusing on their idiosyncratic personas.

Type Two

Type Two, also known as the caring interpersonal type, can be seen as generous, demonstrative, people-pleasing, and possessive. For Twos the primal catastrophe involves a fear of not being loved, of being

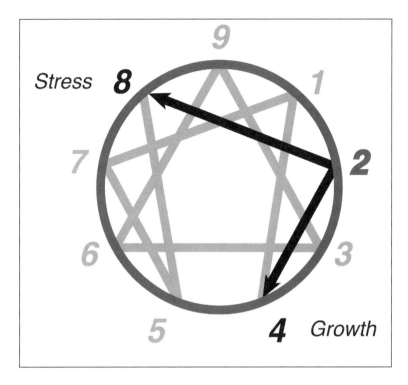

Figure 3.10 Type Two: The Helper. Copyright 2009. The Enneagram Institute. All rights reserved. Used with permission.

unwanted. At times it can go even deeper than that as the person believes that there is no love around, no love in them, and no love in the universe. Twos are consequently motivated to feel loved, to be needed and appreciated, and to do good things for others nearly to a fault to get this love and appreciation.

As caretakers, Twos are constantly thinking of others, anticipating their needs, and meeting these needs so that others will think well of them. Twos are very self-sacrificing and will see to it that others are served first, maintaining a sense of denial about their own needs. Their own needs essentially become meeting the needs of others first. Brian calls this "the boomerang theory of love." They tell themselves, "I will send this love out and if I am needed, I will be loved in return."

As you might expect, Twos have significant boundary problems that adversely impact their ability to sustain healthy and meaningful relations with others. They fail to set appropriate boundaries and limits for themselves, frequently agreeing to take on more than they can really handle. The word "No" doesn't seem part of their vocabulary. Additionally, they disregard others' boundaries, doing things for them that they do not necessarily want done. If there is resistance to the help offered, or others feel crowded by a Two's efforts to help, and there are attempts to establish boundaries, Twos can feel rejected and insecure about the relationship. In the end, their feelings are easily hurt and they fail to understand the perceived rejections because they were "only trying to help."

In general, Twos are looking to be someone's "best friend" so that they can be sought out for assistance or advice or share personal information and become a confidant. They want to feel loved and ensure that others need them. To do this they may act as "martyrs" to anyone's cause or engage in rescuing or enabling behaviors. They can become upset and distressed if they perceive rejection or feel that they are being "left out" or not invited to some social gathering.

At their best, Twos are kind, compassionate, warm hearted, and filled with good will and generosity of spirit. Being genuinely empathic allows healthy Twos to understand another's sorrow and pain, which motivates them to assist and support those in need. Healthy Twos, unlike unhealthy Twos, extend love, support, and assistance without any expectation of being or needing to be loved in return. Integrating Twos, like healthy Fours, become more honest with themselves and discover a lighter side of life as they become more intimate with themselves, losing their sense of shame that impeded personal growth.

Under stressful circumstances that seem beyond their control, Twos tend to perceive their acts of kindness as unappreciated or thwarted, which in turn generates anger that manifests itself in behaviors more reminiscent of average-to-unhealthy Eights. Resentment builds when Twos believe others are taking them for granted or taking advantage of them, and it is during such duress that they act out by becoming egocentric, domineering, controlling of people around them. When under greater stress, disintegrating Twos can become aggressive and threaten to withdraw support.

Twos grow by realizing that they can take care of themselves and others without sacrificing one for the other. They understand that many things in life are reminiscent of the flight attendant's advice in case of emergency to "attend to yourself first before attempting to help those around you." By maintaining love and intimacy with themselves Twos can express their genuine thoughts and feelings, even if those thoughts and feelings are unpleasant or unpopular. This requires self-recognition concerning their feelings, for example, when they are tired, overextended, or lonely. Learning to say "no" without fear of retribution or rejection promotes growth for Twos and allows them to be even more helpful and effective with others.

Habit Control Work With Twos. Habit issues for Type Twos involve nurturing and indirection of behavior. Twos by their very nature are empathic and are often very good at nurturing others but not themselves. The last thing they want is to be perceived by others as selfish and uncaring. The indirection mentioned above for Twos involves caring for others at the expense of themselves. Ultimately, food becomes a source of nurturing as it is not perceived as being particularly selfish. Consequently, it has been our experience that Twos tend to be more prone to being overweight than other personality types. For instance, over the years, David has organized and facilitated a number of weight management groups that employed the RHETI and has found that a disproportionate number of members were Twos than expected based on the general population.

Therapeutically, it is helpful for Twos to appreciate the difference between self-nurturing (nurturing that which is sustainable and ecological) and self-indulgence (getting caught up in the moment of overdoing). Like Nines, as discussed above, Twos have difficulty setting their own agenda and goals because they can be so "other" focused.

Because Twos are the most interpersonally oriented, sometimes the motivation for initiating and empowering change will be based on another person, perhaps a spouse or a lover or someone in their family seeking favors or assistance.

In a similar vein, much of a Type Two's habit behavior will be socially determined. Twos may therefore overeat or smoke primarily because of social issues. They seek and participate in social activities that reinforce eating unhealthy foods (men's or ladies' night out at the dinner buffet) or smoking cigarettes in more socially accepted places (e.g., bars, bowling alleys). It therefore becomes important to examine the person's social issues and social needs and the relationship of these issues/needs to habits.

At times, habit change for Twos requires setting social limits that involve restrictions and at times this can be very uncomfortable and difficult. For instance, not going to the All-You-Can-Eat Buffet or not taking a smoking break with coworkers can make for uncomfortable experiences. As Twos like to "people-please," they may struggle with the notion that their friends or significant others will be upset with them for foregoing activities that are unhealthy. In many ways this is reflective of recommendations to the alcoholic to disconnect from other alcoholics and social events that promote alcohol consumption.

As with Type Nines, we want to deliver the message that "These changes will make you more comfortable." Therefore, in our therapy it is important to help Twos realize that their social nature and their interactions and relationships with others do not have to suffer simply because they are not smoking or not indulging in the smorgasbord with others.

Our therapeutic approaches to Twos are most effective when they are warm, personal, empathetic, and supportive. Twos can be very sensitive to rejection and they tend to be warm and interpersonal with others. If as a therapist you are not warm in return, a Two may feel rejected or disliked. Realize that this approach should not be equated with enabling Twos by being less than genuine or real through warmth and empathy. It is more a matter of meeting them where they are and making them comfortable. At times, conflict in therapy may arise and the issue of rejection and abandonment needs to be addressed accordingly. Walking on eggshells or tip-toeing around the issues is not at all encouraged. In fact, at times, Twos will respond best to more direct feedback, provided it is couched in supportive and caring terms.

Another element that typically requires attention in our therapy with Twos involves boundaries. Twos tend to lack sufficient boundaries, rendering them vulnerable to the manipulation and exploitation of others. By the same token, Twos fail to respect the boundaries of others and can be rather intrusive and needy. It is therefore beneficial to help Twos appreciate reciprocity in relationships.

Twos tend to evaluate their self-esteem through the eyes of others. Their superego message is, "You are okay if you are loved by others and are close to them." As such, they are prone to disappointment and confusion in identity, which enhances the possibility of developing and maintaining unhealthy habits. As therapists, our goal with Twos should also include gaining a sense of individuation whereby the person can

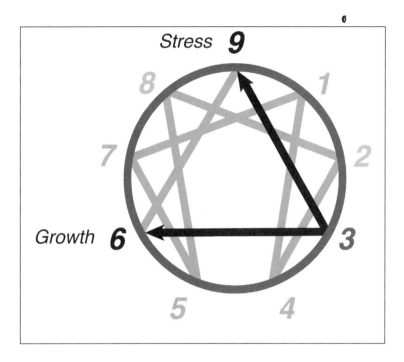

Figure 3.11 Type Three: The Achiever. Copyright 2009. The Enneagram Institute. All rights reserved. Used with permission.

appreciate that they are okay without the approval or acceptance of others. Enhancing their self-esteem and self-reliance will foster the change they want to make to live a healthier and happier life.

Type Three

Sometimes called the performer, the motivator, the success-oriented efficient type, Threes are best known for being admirable, excelling, driven, and image-oriented. The basic fear for Threes is lacking worth or value, and feeling empty or deficient. In sum, it is the fear of failure. To minimize this fear, Threes work diligently to develop themselves, whether physically or mentally, and thrive on setting goals, seeing them through, and seeking recognition and valuation from others for their accomplishments. At times, Threes engage in chameleon-like behavior by changing their goals so as to be the absolute best at whatever seems to be valued by others. When conflicted, Threes can be seen to engage in competitive, self-promoting behavior that can be boastful and grandiose.

Though Type Threes operate on a feeling level and consequently are included in the Feeling Triad, they tend to ignore their feelings, or put them to the side, as they see them get in the way of whatever it is that they intend to accomplish. By denying or ignoring their feelings, Threes are at great risk for burning out and, in the end, accomplishing nothing. This of course is very frightening for Threes and can be a double-edged sword as they maintain an acute awareness of their fear of failure and the potential for "failure" because they pushed themselves too hard and too long.

Threes can be very charismatic, knowing how to put their best foot forward and instill a sense of confidence in others. Above all, Threes are goal directed. They also enjoy sharing their ideas and insights with others, helping them set their own goals, whether it is making money, losing weight, or becoming permanent nonsmokers.

Developmentally, Threes learned in childhood that they are valuable for their accomplishments and self-presentation. They maintain the belief that love comes when they excel at something. Unfortunately, being driven to be the best at whatever they do creates conflicts within their personal and family lives. As expected, intimacy issues are not uncommon as Threes are too busy engaging in goal-oriented behaviors to take time to share intimate moments with others. For unhealthy Threes, intimacy is a diversion or distraction that must be avoided at all costs as it could risk failure and, God forbid, humiliation.

Threes are very image conscious and may work diligently to a fault at staying in excellent physical condition and being well groomed. They want their partner and those close to them to be proud of their accomplishments; consequently, they tend to surround themselves with people whom they believe will appreciate and support them in all their endeavors.

At their best, healthy Threes are excellent communicators, motivational speakers, and promoters of causes they believe in. They excel at "coaching" and building morale and company spirit by inspiring those around them. If there is one distinguishing characteristic of a healthy Three, it is in understanding that life is not a competition. They are passionate about their work and enjoy working with others without needing to outperform their peers. Integrating Threes, like healthy Sixes, release their fear of failure and seek cooperative working relations that serve to benefit the greater good rather than their own ego-driven needs.

Unhealthy or disintegrating Threes drive themselves too hard, become burned out, and engage in "autopilot" behavior much like an average Nine. Under duress, Threes disengage and become passive, losing their focus and drive. They may become depressed and apathetic and no longer enjoy things that are usually pleasurable. Not wanting to hear that they have a problem (which is perceived as a sign of failure), unhealthy Threes become stubborn and resistant to help.

Threes grow by recognizing that it is not necessary to separate their work from their feelings. By living in "the now," being mindful of their feelings, Threes can derive greater pleasure from their work just for the work they do rather than the achievements that feed their egos.

Habit Control Work With Threes. Habit control work for Threes involves elements of competition, emotional detachment, performance, and appearance. Of all the types, Threes are generally considered the most competitive type, not only with others, but with themselves. Tapping into this competitive spirit, provided it tends to be demonstrated in a healthy manner, can be very helpful when addressing habit control for Threes. Reframing habit-control work in ways that captures elements of competition, success, and physical appearance for Threes will enhance their ability to control and manage their unwanted habit. As goal-directed people, Threes will respond well to established goals that will allow them to look better in their eyes and in others' eyes.

When engaging Threes in therapy, it is important and most helpful to remain motivated, positive, and goal oriented. Maintaining goals with the client will also allow Threes to establish a sense of trust and understanding that you are there to help them, not compete with them. At the same time, it will be helpful to teach Threes how to relax, take a break, and minimize the risk of burnout. Threes may become particularly self-destructive when they become overwhelmed and perceive themselves as failing to meet their established goals.

The following is a lighthearted, yet poignant vignette that David frequently shares with his clients to help them reframe their notion of failure:

> A young boy holding a baseball in one hand and a bat resting on his shoulder is determined that today, he will hit the ball. He tosses the ball

in the air, takes a hard and fast swing. Looking to the ground he sees that he missed the ball. "Strike one," he says to himself. Now more determined, he fixes an eye on the ball, the other closed to ensure an accurate swing, throws the ball in the air and takes a second swing. "Strike two," he declares, as he reaches down and picks up the ball. With a deep sigh, he stretches his arm away from him, ball in hand. Knowing this could be his last chance he tosses the ball in the air one final time, fixes his attention on the revolving red stitches and makes a determined swat at the free falling ball. As he completes his swing, nearly toppling over from the forceful rotation, he hears the ball fall to the ground. Placing the bat confidently on his shoulder, he bends over, retrieves the ball, and proudly announces, "I'm one heck of a pitcher."

Ultimately, through our work with Threes we want to help them become more inner directed and authentic with themselves. Authenticity involves being present in a heartfelt way to one's own sense of worth and value, being in touch with feelings without any expectation of success or fear of failure. Because Threes' habits are generally derived from a dysfunctional sense of competition or expectation (real or imagined), it is necessary to help them get in touch with their feelings through some creative endeavor, such as painting, writing, or playing music, that is for their own benefit and enjoyment, with its own inherent value that is not dependent upon the acceptance and kudos of an audience.

Of all the personality types in the Enneagram, though Threes are least likely to meditate, they are the most likely to benefit from it. For Threes, sitting and doing "nothing" is a cardinal sin that makes little sense to their taskmaster ego. Threes must learn that meditating is a far cry from doing nothing, and in fact is likely to be quite challenging for them. In this regard, their willingness to "practice" meditation may be enhanced as they may perceive it as some kind of competition, something to be accomplished. Although this seems counterintuitive, as therapists assisting Threes, given their competitive nature, in this case, the ends (relaxation) justify the means (more competition). When Threes realize that to simply *be* rather than *do* is an accomplishment, they may begin to make therapeutic breakthroughs that have sudden impact for enhancing control over unwanted habits.

As Threes embrace their authenticity, they begin to understand that they are valuable not for what they do or what they've accomplished,

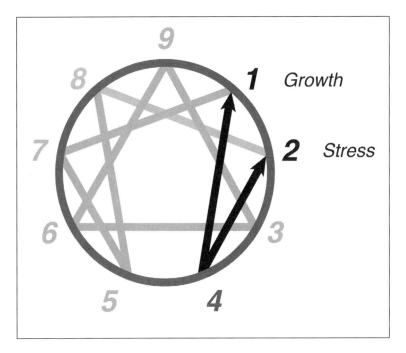

Figure 3.12 Type Four: The Individualist. Copyright 2009. The Enneagram Institute. All rights reserved. Used with permission.

but simply because they exist. This in turn can free them from the habits that seem to control them, particularly those involving "workaholism," which in the end could be the very thing that destroys them.

Type Four

Sometimes called the artist, or the romantic, or the sensitive withdrawn type, Fours are best known for being expressive, dramatic, self-absorbed, and temperamental. The basic fear for Fours is that they will lack a stable identity or sense of personal significance. A secondary fear for Fours is a fear of being flawed or defective in some way that may lead to rejection. Fours are therefore driven to discover themselves and identify their significance through their own special and unique abilities and talents. Their moodiness, self-absorption, and temperamental moods can readily put them at odds with others. Yet when they are creative, self-aware, and emotionally strong, they are valued by others and become inspired to do great things.

Fours tend to identify themselves by their feeling states. As such, their identity can fluctuate, and remain volatile and perhaps unstable as their feelings are very changeable and frequently in flux. Fours are very cognizant of their emotional states and quickly notice when they are upset, anxious, irritable, or happy. They rely on their feelings to help them understand who they are and what their environment is all about.

Fours, as mentioned above, tend to be artistic. They seek out art, poetry, music, and other emotional outlets that they find attractive, because they believe these feelings reveal something about their true identity. They are very motivated to distinguish themselves from others, to stand out in a crowd and let others know that they are *different* and *unique*. By doing so, they are seeking to understand and identify *their own* identity. After all, if in their minds they are not like others, they have truly defined themselves.

Unfortunately, by maintaining such a unique identity, Fours risk feeling alone and misunderstood. Although any of the nine types can feel sad, alone, depressed, or excluded, Fours feel this way frequently, even when there is nothing going on in their lives to substantiate such feelings.

Fours essentially want to express their individuality and surround themselves with self-created beauty that puts their own stamp on their environment. At the same time, they may withdraw, protecting their vulnerabilities, knowing they are "different," all the while seeking and desiring a "rescuer" who will support and understand them.

High-functioning Fours are sensitive to others, especially their feelings, and typically enjoy exchanging personal life experiences. They can be excellent listeners, though this at times is masked by the intensity of drama and self-absorbed emotions that keep others at a distance. They can be very temperamental and moody, leaving others with a feeling that they must "walk on eggshells" or survive the rollercoaster ride of emotional volatility that characterizes their existence. Fours maintain a sense of perpetual victimization and have difficulty shifting from this perspective to one of a "survivor." They tend to focus on past pains and emotional suffering rather than working through those hurts in productive ways that involve a process of therapeutic forgiveness.

At their best, Fours are true to themselves and others, looking very much like healthy Ones as they become involved in matters that extend beyond themselves. They are emotionally honest and unafraid of expressing their feelings to anyone. They invite others to reveal themselves, the good, the bad, and the ugly. When functioning well, Fours help others feel comfortable in their own skin and do so with a sense of gentleness, tact, and discretion. Highly functioning Fours are very creative and inspired by and in tune with the ever-changing world around them.

When under stress, Fours disintegrate by defending their hurt feelings and by gaining attention from others through their victimization, despite awareness on some level that this behavior likely drives others away. Dysfunctional Fours can become possessive of loved ones, not wanting them to be out of their sight, much like lower-functioning Twos. An exaggerated example of a Type Four, though clearly hitting the mark, is the character portrayed by Glenn Close in the film *Fatal Attraction.*

Fours grow by recognizing that despite painful and difficult life experiences, they can put these experiences behind them. These disappointing, painful, perhaps traumatic events don't have to haunt them forever. Healthy fours understand that, just as the wake of a boat won't ever steer the course of the boat, their past does not have to have direct influence on their current or future experiences.

Habit Control Work With Fours. For Type Fours, the habit issues involve feelings, moods, fantasy, and self-absorption. As individualists, Fours can be very mood oriented, as their primary focus tends to be their feelings and what their feelings tell them about their environment, which in turn ultimately guides their behavior. How they feel will have a direct and significant impact on how they eat, drink, or smoke, as this behavior, though destructive, will be rationalized one way or the other according to their feelings.

Fours will, for instance, justify their binging, smoking, or drinking by reference to their suffering, anxiety, and emotional pain. It is not uncommon for them to assert that binging would be expected in certain circumstances because they feel so bad. Medication, alcohol, and illicit substances are rationalized as necessities for controlling certain feelings and emotional discomfort.

One of David's former female clients, Claire, a 56-year-old, with an identified personality type of Four with a Three wing (also known as the Aristocrat), would frequently start her therapy session off by reviewing her week of pain and suffering at the hands of her unappreciative adult children who neglect and abandon her whenever she calls or visits them. The pained week-in-review was predictably followed by justification for her continued misuse of clonazepam, a frequently prescribed psychotropic medication for anxiety disorders, and ice cream binges that on occasion amounted to a half-gallon in one sitting.

Therapeutically, Fours want to be seen as unique and special and in touch with a full range of feelings. Behavioral therapy that focuses on concrete objectives with measured outcomes is as uncomfortable for Fours as Psychodrama is for Fives. Dr. Phil, for instance, would likely frighten a Four right off the stage and have her running to the dressing room before he could even ask, "Is that working for you?" Therapy should therefore allow ample opportunity to process feelings, though this should be done judiciously, as it could be overused and detract from the habit-control work that needs to be done.

When distraught, Fours tend to become withdrawn, drowning in their feelings, lost in fantasy, and being extremely unproductive. It is essential that Fours engage in treatment on levels that surpass emotional processing so that they can become more functional and active.

Reminding Fours that "feelings are not facts" and that they do not necessarily provide accurate information about others' motivations or feelings can be helpful. Though at times difficult for the therapist, given the risk of inflicting a narcissistic wound, it will be necessary to address their fantasy life and help them align this with the reality of their life. Having creative goals and working toward "life dreams" is admirable and wonderful. Procrastinating or fantasizing about attaining these goals without action or effort is self-defeating. Likewise, when Fours maintain a sense of entitlement, believing their talents and abilities are extraordinarily unique and special will only continue to swell a swollen head, that is sure to accomplish little to nothing other than frustration and irritability over the sense that others fail to appreciate them.

Fours, like Threes, need an occasional "reality check." As therapists, we encourage them to seek friends who can be honest and accurate. People who appreciate their genuine good and creative qualities and talents as well as identify areas that could use improvement will offer growth opportunities for Fours in ways that minimize additional conflict and distress. Of course this will largely depend on the health of the individual and her capacity to accept direct and honest feedback.

Fantasy life, in particular, can be destructive for Fours, as their grandiose tendencies involve an overestimation of their true talents and abilities. This leads to ridicule and rejection from others who have heard the exaggerated stories more times than they care to count. This in turn reinforces isolation and alienation and also fosters rejection of any offered assistance from others, which leaves Fours vulnerable for engaging in unhealthy and unwanted habits.

Therapeutic interventions with Fours are most effective when coupled with a message that their essence is not in any creative process, but simply in who they are. Self-esteem work is generally necessary so that Fours can appreciate that there is nothing "wrong" with them, that they do not need "rescuing, " and they are as good as everyone else, just different, as we all are.

It may also be necessary to include forgiveness in the therapeutic process with Fours. Though at times they may find creative inspiration through their painful life experiences, they may hold onto these experiences in ways that promote self-destructive habits. When this is the case, forgiveness can be freeing for Fours as they recognize and appreciate that pain and suffering have allowed them to become the person they are with all of their wonderful talents, abilities, and flaws.

The Thinking Triad

The Thinking Triad, also known as "The Head Center," is comprised of Types Five, Six, and Seven. For this triad, anxiety is the primary emotion behind the personality. Fives have anxiety about the outer world and their capacity to cope with it; Sixes, being the most anxious of all the types, are doubtful about themselves; and Sevens have anxiety about their inner world. For this triad, the primary theme is seeking security and support. Fives seek security by detaching and turning to the world of imagination; Sixes seek support from others and ideas and suggestions others offer; and Sevens aren't quite sure where or how to find security, so they do a little bit of everything.

Type Five

Fives are known for being intense and cerebral. They are focused, observant, curious, insightful, and studious. They are best known for

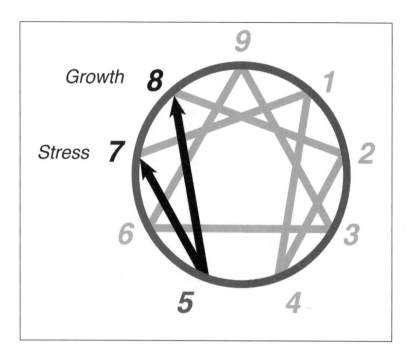

Figure 3.13 Type Five: The Investigator. Copyright 2009. The Enneagram Institute. All rights reserved. Used with permission.

being perceptive, innovative, secretive, and isolated. They compensate for their primary anxiety, of being useless and helpless, by attempting to acquire knowledge and understanding all that they can about the environment they live in. They live by the maxim "knowledge is power." Others find them difficult and challenging to relate to when they become detached, preoccupied, and isolated. However, it is their visionary and pioneering ideas that allow them to grow and attract others to them.

Fives seem to need more privacy than most people, and they can become somewhat isolative living the life of a minimalist. Said differently, Fives could be considered "loners" and "misfits." Boredom is not usually a concern for Fives, as they always have their imagination to rely on. At times, however, they may become so engrossed in their own fantasies and imagination that they fail to consider their environment, or even neglect to take care of themselves. For instance, they may become so involved in a project, work, or reading that they are often late for meetings or forget them altogether.

Though prone to isolation, this is not necessarily preferred by Fives. Quite the contrary, Fives are drawn to individuals who share similar intellectual pursuits or anyone willing to listen to them. Typically, Fives are odd, quirky, and socially awkward, making it less likely that they will be gregarious extroverts.

At their best, Fives appreciate the price paid for their social isolation and risk getting in touch with themselves by becoming more grounded in their bodies and their life energy. They become more confident in their abilities to take on leadership roles, manifesting the confidence of a healthy Eight. When moving toward a level of integration, Fives recognize that others seek them out as a source of wisdom, knowledge, and quiet strength.

When distressed, Fives look like average Sevens. Hyperactive and scattered behaviors become more the norm for a disintegrating Five, who also becomes rather hyperverbal and impulsive. They tend to be nervous and high strung when there isn't an outlet for their nervous energy.

Fives grow by recognizing that confidence comes from putting themselves out in the real world, among other people, rather than through mastering some intellectual curiosity. They naturally derive confidence from their well-developed minds; however, growth occurs for Fives when they develop a deeper and more meaningful relationship with their bodies and through the expression of feelings. Remember, Fives are included within the Thinking Triad and, although they feel things deeply, they struggle with expressing their feelings to others in a genuine manner. Developing trust in their relationships, feeling more comfortable with sharing their feelings, and identifying with their feelings will serve as the key that unlocks the door for them to appreciate their true potential.

Habit Control Work With Fives. Habit issues for Type Five personalities involve minimization. In essence, for Fives, the less they need, the less they ask of people; and the less they ask of people, the less people ask of them. Consequently, the world will require little from them, and this will minimize any potential conflict in life, at least for Fives.

Minimization is a breeding ground for poor habits. Because Fives are more in touch with their intellect than with their physical well-being, the body suffers when they engage in unhealthy habits. Fives tend to avoid exercise or maintaining good dietary habits, as their predominant focus is on their mind, not their body. Sitting in front of a computer for hours on end, expanding the intellect while grazing on fast food, high-carbohydrate food, soft drinks, and chain-smoking captures the stereotypical image of a Type Five.

One of David's clients, J.D., was a 43-year-old self-employed computer programmer who had been isolating himself in a home office, chain-smoking, and living on fast-food burgers and fries for several years. His depression and anxiety had exacerbated to the degree that he would only leave his home when absolutely necessary, and it was rarely absolutely necessary. Exercise was as foreign to J.D. as kerning is to most of us. Fives epitomize the information and technology age and are constantly yearning to learn more through their own investigative efforts. It is therefore helpful, as it was in J.D.'s case, to provide Fives with information that is accurate and acquired from a reliable source.

Knowing J.D. was either going to gather more information about computers or other personally intellectually curious subjects, David took advantage of J.D.'s inquisitive nature and provided him with an ample supply of data concerning cigarette smoking. Like most Fives, J.D. was likely to look at the information with a critical and skeptical eye, so David ensured that all of the information was accurate, from reliable sources (such as those offered throughout this text), and not simply based on scare tactics, poorly controlled studies, or unreliable information. Otherwise, as a therapist, David would lose credibility in J.D.'s eyes, not to mention his respect.

Additional interventions were incorporated into J.D.'s therapy, though the provision of information was crucial for enhancing the likelihood that J.D. would become a permanent nonsmoker. Therefore, whenever you are working with a Type Five personality, offer them as much information as you can, without concern of overwhelming them, as they will consume this data which in the end could be the primary influence on habit change.

As Fives tend to be cerebral, it is also important in our therapeutic efforts with them to foster interactions with others. Helping them reach out to others to enhance connectedness will enable them to grow as individuals and appreciate that they can relate to others, understanding that they do not need to retreat into the inner sanctum of their minds. We find it very beneficial to encourage Fives to teach others what they learn through the material we provide them. This likely comes more natural to them and, as therapists, we can capitalize on their "intellectual

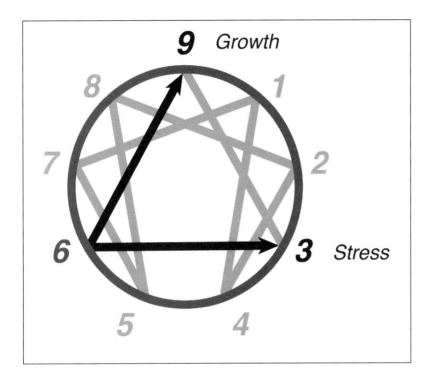

Figure 3.14 Type Six: The Loyalist. Copyright 2009. The Enneagram Institute. All rights reserved. Used with permission.

prowess" to facilitate interpersonal relationships. Furthermore, having them share this information affirms their desire to change unwanted behaviors and remain motivated to become permanent nonsmokers and/or permanently fit and trim.

Type Six

Sixes are best known for being committed. They are engaging, responsible, anxious, and suspicious. They operate on the basic fear that they will be alone, without support and guidance. They are generally hard working, reliable, vigilant, persevering, cautious, and anxious. They can be pessimistic, doubtful, negativistic and reactive, and at their worst may be suspicious and blaming. Others find them attractive and appealing because they can be cooperative, funny, affectionate, and grounded.

Sixes epitomize the hard-working and industrious person who desires to create a stable, safe environment where everyone can work together. They tend to be attentive to details and are quite skilled at anticipating problems before they become overwhelming and unmanageable. Sixes like the notion that they can belong to a group, but they are by no means "group people."

Unfortunately, Sixes tend to stew in a state of anxiety. If there is nothing to worry about you can be sure the Six will find something to worry about. Generally cautious and careful in their dealings with others, they are ever mindful of the people that can be trusted who will be on their side when the going gets tough. Sixes will also rely on a sense of humor to engage people and get their attention and approval. They thrive in social situations in which they are familiar with the people around them; but situations in which they are surrounded by strangers, where there are too many unknowns, leave them unsurefooted.

Lacking self-confidence, Sixes frequently look outside of themselves to other sources of support and experience. For instance, they may seek a mentor or authority figure who can guide them. They prefer predictability to spontaneity and desire reassurances like the daily affirmations of Al Franken's fictitious self-help guru, Stuart Smalley, *"I'm good enough; I'm smart enough; and doggone it, people like me!"*

More than anything else, Sixes desire a sense of peace and inner quiet that allows them to more accurately perceive and respond to their environment. Their hypervigilance precludes clear thinking and effective planning to address whatever challenge may be confronting them.

When functioning well, Sixes look like Healthy Nines. They are engaging, playful, friendly, and gain a greater understanding and acceptance of life's ups and downs. Integrating Sixes are not riddled with a sense of constant dread and anxiety. They are free to let their minds rest and enjoy peaceful, quiet moments.

At their worst, they disintegrate into Average Threes, reacting with self-doubt, engaging in frantic efforts to minimize their anxiety by working harder, and becoming more task oriented. They deny their feeling states and become preoccupied with accomplishing tasks and goals, some of which look like nothing more than "busy work" that in the end may not accomplish much of anything.

Growth is appreciated for Sixes when they realize that security comes from within. When sixes understand that all of the external resources that have been put in place, including financial security, good friends, and loving family members, will always guarantee security or success, they begin to grow. Life is unpredictable and bad things do happen to good people. As Riso and Hudson note in *Discovering Your Personality Type*, "Sixes will know firsthand the value of discovering their inner resources when they take time to relax their constant vigilance and find faith in themselves" (p. 144).

Habit Control Work With Sixes. Habit control issues for Sixes primarily involve elements of anxiety, reactivity, authority figures, and loyalty. Because anxiety is such a central issue to the Six, anxiety is generally the root cause of the unwanted habit. Anything to deaden, dampen, or manage the anxiety is fair game for Sixes, whether it involves smoking, alcohol consumption, or eating.

Sixes also tend to be very reactive, scanning their environment and at the ready to respond to any perceived threat. To minimize their skepticism, it is important that, as therapists, we be "up front" with Sixes, instilling a sense of trust through our commitment and consistency. We also need to be prepared to reassure Sixes, as they lack confidence and trust in their own abilities and will frequently seek approval and acceptance of others before committing to anything.

Sixes seek feedback from authority figures, so it is not uncommon for them to do so during therapy sessions. A seasoned therapist, however, will be on the watch for a counterphobic reaction from Sixes, as they are prone to both positive and negative transference. Should they misinterpret the therapist as being unjust or unwise, feelings of doubt could readily erupt into rebellion against or rejection of the therapist. Helping them understand that no relationship will *always* provide perfect guidance and support is a necessary part of treatment with Sixes. Otherwise, their doubt and mistrust will continue to plague them time and time again.

Therapists can capitalize on Sixes' sense of loyalty by encouraging them to find a partner or a group that shares a common goal of changing an unwanted behavior. Exercising with others, attending health-focused seminars, and joining a gym could be very therapeutic for Sixes because they have an excellent capacity to work for the greater good of all.

Sixes, like Fives also benefit from information, though information overload and inconsistent data could generate additional anxiety, which must be minimized and avoided if at all possible. Therefore, providing Sixes with "just the facts" that can be readily backed up and supported through some expert treatise, so to speak, could be helpful.

Despite their loyalty, reliability, and sense of seriousness about responsibility, Sixes can be indecisive. They are prone to "yes, but" themselves because they fear making commitments at times, concerned that they may make a "mistake." Consequently, self-affirmation, enhanced self-esteem, and self-reliance that facilitate belief in their own capacities are principal components of therapy with Sixes. Hypnotherapy that includes self-affirming statements as well as opportunities to imagine and create success can reinforce the fact that the source of the support that Sixes need is within themselves.

Type Seven

Also known as the busy, fun-loving type, Sevens are spontaneous, versatile, acquisitive, scattered, and excessive. The basic fear driving Sevens is the fear of being trapped in pain, of being confined and deprived. Sevens are spontaneous, curious, optimistic, outgoing, and adventurous. At the same time, they can be scattered, distracted, restless, and impatient. At times, their relationships are conflicted because they can be irresponsible, demanding, and excessive. When doing well, we see Sevens who are appreciative, grateful, passionate, and accomplished.

Sevens are probably the most enthusiastic, spontaneous, and extroverted of all the types. They are socialites who thrive on having a full calendar of things to do and people to be with. They tend to be very vivacious people who do not sit still for very long as there is always something to do that could be fun and exciting. As Riso and Hudson point out, "Sevens want to try everything at least twice: once to see what it is like, and the second time to see if they liked it the first time!"

Though outwardly they may not present as a bundle of nerves, in reality Sevens are fleeing from their anxieties by engaging in activities that distract them from their fears. They believe that living a life that is exciting and adventurous will thwart the internalized anxiety that in

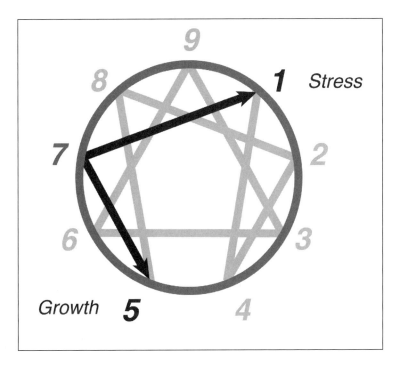

Figure 3.15 Type Seven: The Enthusiast. Copyright 2009. The Enneagram Institute. All rights reserved. Used with permission.

the meantime is still eating them up and in some ways preventing them from living up to their fullest potential. In private, Sevens struggle with loneliness, depression, and self-doubt. They have a sense that no one will take them seriously because of their spontaneous and childlike demeanor. Because they are worried that they may never get what they really want out of life, they settle for other pleasures and vices that they hope will make them happy in the interim.

Unhealthy Sevens disintegrate in ways so that they resemble Average Ones. When under duress, Sevens become scattered and distracted, leaving them so frustrated that they begin to doubt their abilities to accomplish much of anything. This, in turn, leads them in the direction of disintegration, where they forcefully impose order and self-control only to become frustrated, impatient, and irritable. Nothing seems to go their way, so they become harsh and critical of others, much like an unstable Type One.

At their best, Healthy Sevens integrate into Healthy Fives. Their minds become quiet, clear, and focused. They are less scattered, disorganized, and inefficient. The notion of being bored becomes foreign to them as they are able to become more absorbed in the moment instead of distracted by all the things they think they want to do that will give them a sense of purpose and excitement.

Habit Control Work With Sevens. Habit issues for Sevens include the need for constant stimulation, avoidance of pain, and escapism. They are prone to abuse drugs and alcohol to avoid the emotional pain they fear. Their escapism allows them to avoid pain in the present, though much of the emotional pain they try to numb is associated with past traumas and fear of things yet to happen.

Sevens seek constant stimulation to keep themselves distracted from any source of pain that may leave them uncomfortable. As such, they are prone to abusing amphetamines like cocaine, crank, crack, and crystal meth. Of course, nicotine dependence and overeating behaviors are common for Sevens when they are unhealthy or reacting to stress that they find unmanageable. Regardless of the substance used, the price paid (physical, psychological, social, financial, etc.) exceeds that which the individual will experience simply by learning to manage the stress in more productive manners.

Through their avoidance, need for constant stimulation, and impatience, Sevens can readily engage in impulsive behaviors. Although they want to acquire knowledge and skills, they tend to cut corners, relying upon a false sense of bravado and charm and risk being perceived by others as superficial. Helping Sevens "slow down" and "live in the moment" will allow them to appreciate how they are running away from their own lives and from opportunities for personal growth.

If you have experience working with substance abusers, you have no doubt appreciated how the cognitive, emotional, and interpersonal skills of addicts are delayed and less mature than their non-abusing peers. Rather than develop effective coping skills to manage life's difficulties, addicts rely on drugs and/or alcohol to escape personal challenges and remain "stuck" at a developmental level that may be more consistent with adolescence. It therefore is important to consider the emotional maturity of the client and ensure that our expectations do not exceed their capacity to follow through with therapeutic recommendations. At times, they will be irrational, illogical, defensive, and unreceptive to suggestions that for most clients make sense and are readily embraced.

An orientation toward the future can be frightening for Sevens, particularly when they believe that they may be depriving themselves of something, like a piece of cake or a cigarette. Despite this irrational perception, we, as therapists, can help Sevens understand how engaging in their unhealthy behavior or habit ultimately deprives them of the benefits of better health, a more fit and trim body, and energy that allows them to engage in life's adventures. Sevens enjoy being active contributors in their world. They would rather make the food than eat it, or create the movie than watch it. Therapy, therefore, must be positive, encouraging, and action-oriented, with an ample dose of relaxation and meditation interjected to help Sevens *slow down* and *smell the roses*.

Sevens benefit from treatment that is predominantly behavioral and upbeat. Learning to manage pain in healthier and more productive ways is also crucial for Sevens if they are to manage their unwanted habits. Because hypnosis is a passive intervention, it can be a hard sell for many Sevens. However, in our opinion, this is not a valid excuse for dismissing it entirely. In fact, if Sevens understand how they "create" their own experience during hypnosis, and that trance work really involves helping them get in touch with their unconscious mind to access and mobilize their own resources, Sevens may be more receptive to the notion of hypnosis. It may also be helpful for them to understand how hypnosis can be "fun and exciting" as they can learn to experience a number of sensations and perceptions that can minimize and control pain.

CONCLUSION

In this chapter, we introduced you to the Enneagram of Personality Types and more specifically the Riso-Hudson Enneagram Type Indicator, a self-administered forced-choice personality inventory that helps us understand why we have conflicts with certain people, yet with others we may feel an instant, and perhaps longstanding, bond or connectedness. When used properly, the Enneagram offers valuable data about our clients that help facilitate and individualize treatment of unwanted habits.

Though a complicated tool, understanding each personality type including the levels of development, direction of integration and disintegration, and the wings of each type allows client and therapist alike to gain a greater appreciation of the factors that contribute to habit development and maintenance and the keys for unlocking these unwanted behaviors.

All nine personality types were reviewed and identified according to their respective triad (Feeling, Instinctive, Thinking) and relevant habit-control treatment issues were discussed for each type.

Things to Do

1. Take the full RHETI and identify assets and abilities that can enhance your work with your clients based on a greater understanding of yourself.
2. Identify other Personality Types that may be challenging for you to work with and generate your plan for minimizing countertransference reactions that could interfere with treatment and progress.
3. Ask one of your clients to take the full RHETI and develop a treatment plan for habit control based on their inventory results.

Teach Them and Let Them Lead the Way

Many of life's failures are people who did not realize how close to success they were when they gave up.

—*Thomas Edison*

4

Soliciting Reasons for Change: Why Now?

It is not the strongest of the species that survives, nor the most intelligent, but the one most responsive to change.

—Charles Darwin

In the previous chapter we reviewed the Enneagram and its utility for establishing a treatment plan for eliminating unwanted behaviors. In many ways, the Enneagram serves as a framework for understanding our clients' underlying attitudes and perceptions of themselves and their environment, as well as providing valuable insight regarding their personality, relationships with others, typical patterns of behavior (healthy and dysfunctional), guidance with enhancing personal growth and, more specifically, greater control over unwanted habits.

In this chapter we address the process of helping people eliminate unwanted habits through strategic, and at times preordained, questions that purposefully elicit and suggest a process of change consistent with the client's motivation and attitudes. As you will see, it is not only the question asked that is relevant, but *how* the question is posed that is of significance. By carefully tending to a client's language, we can solicit responses and carefully reframe the client's words and thoughts in ways that promote the probability of productive change. This approach, along with other carefully considered and timely interventions, borrows heavily from the Solution Focused and/or Strategic Therapy movement, which emphasizes client strengths and past successes to maximize therapeutic possibilities while minimizing a rearview-mirror perspective that analyzes and scrutinizes past failures or shortcomings.

Solution Focused Therapy interventions are built on the notion that most people's solutions to the problems confronting them are present and available, though not quite accessed and mobilized efficiently. Rather than dwell on the presenting problem, which only creates *more of the same,* we remain mindful of Albert Einstein's definition of insanity—doing the same thing over and over again and expecting different results. We help our clients recognize and examine the exceptions to the presenting problem, in addition to helping them reframe their experience and thought processes in ways that promote effective and permanent solutions for their unwanted behaviors. For example, rather than encourage our clients to simply list all of the precipitants of a binge episode or the distressful events that lead to chain smoking (e.g., boredom, fast-food commercial, loneliness), we may ask them about times when they opted *not* to binge *despite* prime opportunities for doing so, or when they were able to refrain from lighting up that first cigarette during stressful experiences. Ultimately, we are looking for any exceptions to the rule, for therein may lie a solution, or perhaps part of a solution, to the problem.

In our quest to solicit reasons for change, it is important to listen to the language of the client and re-tool it or rephrase it when necessary. We may reframe the client's statements in subtle but powerful ways, as the words our clients use define them and their perspective on themselves and their lives. Without conscious awareness, many people speak in negative terms when identifying therapeutic treatment goals. For instance, a client may say, "As John the permanent nonsmoker, I will not be so tired or physically exhausted." Though there is nothing inherently wrong with this comment, we may take the opportunity to rephrase it a bit and offer the following suggestion: "As John, a permanent nonsmoker, I will have increased energy and more endurance."

We could even take it a step further to make it more concrete, promoting an expectation of change (more on this in chapter 8, vis-à-vis hypnosis) that is more measurable and experienced on a number of sensory levels. For example, we may add to the above sentence, "I will be able to come home after a day's work and play with my kids, or mow the lawn, or go for a walk or work out at the gym." In doing so, not only have we helped the client reframe his initial statement from a negative "I will not _____" to a positive "I will _____," we have also encouraged him to identify the benefits of changing his behavior to eliminate the unwanted habit.

Rather than *give* them the reasons for changing their unwanted behavior, we *solicit* that information from them. So, if for instance someone indicates that one of the reasons for not smoking or for dieting and exercising is to "be more active," we could ask, "Being more active to do what?" Or if someone says, "I would be able to travel more," again, we could counter with a question that concretizes this goal: "Where would you go? What kind of traveling would you do?"

Provided you don't overkill the situation with too many questions that ultimately frustrate your client, you could go one step further after she responds to your last question. If the client said, "I would be more active by exercising or gardening," you could follow this statement by asking, "How often do you think you would exercise? What kind of exercising would you do? Where would you exercise? When do you think you would be ready to exercise?"

By helping the client expound the reasons for becoming a non-smoker or permanently fit individual, we help foster a sense of momentum and excitement that motivates him to initiate the change that is needed in his life.

As you will see in chapter 8, on hypnosis, one essential element of habit control therapy is the notion of presupposition. The presupposition in the preceding situations is that the person *will become* the permanent nonsmoker, the permanently slim, fit, and healthy person. During our sessions, we frequently use these words with the patient and repeat such phrases as, "So, as Jim the permanent nonsmoker, you will _____." This serves as the mantra for the therapeutic work as we build this expectation, much as we do when utilizing other interventions that set the stage for habit control.

We also write these reasons down on a piece of paper for the client so that she or he has this information to refer to later and so this important message doesn't get lost in the course of the therapy session.

ELICITING REASONS FOR CHANGE

In chapter 2 we discussed Julian Rotter's Social Learning Theory and more specifically the distinction between internal and external locus of control. We noted how individuals with a high *internal locus of control* (or "internals") maintain that events occur in direct relation to their own behavior and actions. Those with a high *external locus of control* (or "externals") believe that powerful others, fate, and/or chance primarily determine outcomes and events. We also mentioned how internals have better control of their behavior and are more likely to attempt to influence other people than are externals. Internals are more likely to assume that their efforts will be successful.

Although we cannot necessarily influence people to the degree that we can procedurally convert an external to an internal, we believe that we can influence or at the very least modify an external's mindset in ways that can, if even briefly, reflect the perspective maintained by internals. Knowing that internals are also internally driven and motivated (versus driven and motivated by external means, for example, to please others) and that such motivation tends to produce longer-lasting or, if you will, permanent change, it stands to reason that fostering internal reasons for change will be far more effective for most people than promoting external reasons for change.

Some clients may readily offer the reasons for ending their unwanted habits. Some come with a list in hand that they have been carrying with them, hoping to gain momentum on their goals. Others may offer vague reasons or reasons that are completely externally motivated, like the teenager whose mother wants him to quit smoking or the overweight housewife whose husband has been creating more stress through critical and belittling comments.

Regardless of whether your client presents a list of reasons for change or not, we recommend that you ensure that health, appearance, logistics, financial benefits, and improved physical and mental abilities are reviewed during the earlier phase of treatment as reasons for seeking change. These reasons are universal when it comes to changing unwanted habits and, in fact, we have found that they serve as an effective means of developing a psychotherapy treatment plan that will likely suffice for any third-party payer requiring quantifiable outcomes for the treatment of many conditions.

Improved health is generally a given when it comes to becoming a permanent nonsmoker or permanently fit and trim individual. Some people may have a particular disease or diseases in mind that they wish to prevent. This can be particularly relevant for the individual who has had a family member who may have suffered from some unwanted disease or ailment such as chronic obstructive pulmonary disease, cancer, or cerebrovascular disease.

Two primary health issues that we address with our clients are freedom from illness and improved health that promotes greater levels of energy and vitality. For many of our clients, their families can serve as reasons for improving their health and minimizing the risk of disease. For parents with young children, a healthier life can permit greater levels of participation in family activities such as hiking, sports, and active play that, as any of us who are parents know, can be physically fatiguing. One of David's clients identified playing with her kids at the community pool and walking on the beach as reasons for becoming permanently fit and trim. She had just returned from vacation at the Outer Banks and was frustrated with not being able to participate in activities with her children or walking along the beach with her husband because her hips and knees hurt because of her excessive weight. As you will see in chapter 8, we apply hypnotic interventions to enhance commitment to change by including personal images like this in addition to other information that is relevant for the individual.

For some clients, identifying specific fitness goals can be motivating. Reduced blood pressure and resting pulse rate, weight loss, gains in strength and flexibility, or improved athletic performance such as walking or running in a 5K or 10K race can serve as additional goals or motivators that allow people to remain committed to a healthier lifestyle.

Appearance can be a very important factor for some people wanting to change unwanted habits. Some find this a very reasonable and acceptable goal, whereas other clients may feel a sense of shame if they believe appearance is the predominant reason for changing, especially if that change involves weight loss. These folks struggle with believing that they (and others) should accept themselves as they are regardless of the size of their bodies. In their minds losing weight may seem like "giving in" to a societal standard that just doesn't seem worth the effort. Unfortunately, this perspective can be self-defeating on many levels. In these cases, we want to let people know that it is okay to identify appearance as a reason for changing and that doing so doesn't need to signify raising a white flag of surrender.

We agree that they and others should indeed accept themselves for who they are regardless of the size or shape of their bodies. It should be noted that we do not believe that interpreting this perception as resistance or rationalization for not changing is beneficial or helpful in any way. At the same time, like a different haircut or wearing new clothes, they can be proud of their appearance and of finding ways to enhance it while improving health and fitness in addition to other reasons reviewed below.

Taking it a step further, if necessary, we will review with our clients the difference between self-esteem and confidence. Believing and reinforcing the thought that losing weight, in particular, will enhance their self-worth or self-esteem can lead to a slippery slope indeed. We want to avoid any perception that body size should be equated with self-worth. Establishing an understanding that they may have improved confidence and feel better about themselves because of the things they are able to do is a more effective means of enhancing motivation and maintaining a level of motivation for change.

There are also certain logistics that should be considered when identifying reasons for changing unwanted behavior. For instance, being able to work without interruption as a permanent nonsmoker or going certain places that may otherwise be physically challenging or precluded because it is a nonsmoking establishment may be motivational for some clients. For smokers, having clothes or a home that won't reek of the stale scent of cigarettes can be very motivational. If not for themselves, becoming a nonsmoker is usually a welcome change for nonsmoking family members who are more sensitive to eau-d'ashtray.

Financially, it makes sense to quit smoking or minimize frequent trips to fast-food restaurants. Though one of David's clients argued that living a healthier lifestyle is more expensive, as high-caloric, simple-carbohydrate foods are cheaper and joining a fitness facility or purchasing exercise equipment can be pricey. Although agreeing in principle to some extent, David countered this gentleman's observations with noting the cost of medication and other medical expenses, and the fact that, despite their "deals," the cost of fast-food dining tends to add up, like the calories of a supersized meal.

Finally, when considering goals for habit control, we encourage our clients to consider how implementing desired change can lead to improved skills and abilities. Some activities simply require less effort and are more recreational when our bodies are fit. Whereas most of these activities involve some level of physical exertion, others, such as playing a guitar or other musical instrument, or even driving a car or sitting in a theatre seat, require little to no physical effort, yet would be more enjoyable if a person weren't overweight or huffing and puffing from the effects of cigarette smoking.

Eliciting the Reasons

It is one thing to identify reasons that support and motivate change, but quite another to elicit them from our clients in ways that allow them to process and get in touch with these reasons. This step isn't just an exercise in futility, for, as you will see, this information not only provides additional information regarding how unwanted behaviors are maintained, but also offers relevant information that leads to effective interventions, including hypnosis, energy psychology, and Emotional Freedom Techniques (EFT).

We have identified four primary areas to consider when eliciting change from our clients: emotional, physical, logistical, and personal. The first, and perhaps the most important, is the emotional element. At times, people encounter difficulty accessing, identifying, or even processing emotions when we ask them to consider the feelings that promote or maintain the unwanted behavior. When we encounter these individuals, we offer them examples of possible uncomfortable emotional states they may experience that enhance the probability that they will engage in an unwanted behavior, whether that is smoking or overeating. For instance, we may have them consider stress, feelings of emptiness, loneliness, despair, or hopelessness (to name only a few) when they smoke, overeat, or simply eat when they aren't hungry. With the last example, we will suggest to them that they may be engaging in automatic, seemingly unconscious behavior when they open the refrigerator seeking something to eat when the body isn't physiologically telling them that this is what they need to do. We then explore the notion of how they "narcotize" by numbing themselves to uncomfortable feelings or to thoughts that may lead to uncomfortable feelings.

Emotional reasons can be based on current or recent life predicaments or learned responses to a history of trauma, feelings of abandonment, fear of failure, or other irrational thought patterns spun from years of self-defeating beliefs. These are issues that you can expand upon that should have been captured in the initial data-gathering sessions and have likely been supplemented by the results of Enneagram testing, if that was completed.

There are also physiological reasons to consider when eliciting reasons for change from clients. We will address this in greater detail in the chapters on hypnosis (9), energy psychology, and EFT (11) when we discuss the addictive nature of unwanted habits and the importance of dealing with withdrawal and physical discomfort.

Logistical reasons involve marking out time and rewarding the self during these periods. A number of clients seeking help with habit control mark out time by smoking or taking snack breaks through the day. This time is identified as a time to relax, time to take a break from work or some task, whether it is completed or not. In essence, the behavior is used as a marker to clarify the different phases or stages of what people are doing or to indicate that something is beginning or something has been completed. Logistical reasons can also involve a sense of deserved reward (whether realistic or not) or positive re-inforcement.

Part of this marking out of time may also be a way of relaxing, a self-imposed time-out from the annoyance of the day, if you will. Sometimes people say, "I like to smoke," and we may respond by asking, "What is it that you like about smoking?" Occasionally we hear, "Well, I get to call a time-out, give myself some space, sit back, take some deep breaths, relax." We then reinforce this notion but with parenthetic editing: "That's great that you take time out from the stress of your day like that. More people should do it too. Perhaps you could take this break without cigarettes."

Frequently, part of the logistics of cigarette smoking involves a conditioned association with something else, whether it is coffee, driving in the car, working at the computer, or being with other smokers. Ultimately our goal is to help people engage in these activities without cigarettes. In these situations, however, over time, people associate certain activities or behaviors with smoking. Smoking becomes a marker or cue for this relaxed state to occur during these moments. As you can probably see by now, it is important to elicit the reasons for the unwanted behavior because it allows us to determine what is important for the person versus what is just an association with or an artifact of smoking.

In chapter 2 we discussed the importance of gathering comprehensive historical information about our clients. This information is relevant on many levels and is particularly beneficial for soliciting reasons for behavioral change. Some clients may have histories rich with reasons that habits developed and likewise rich with reasons for wanting (and not wanting) to change particular behaviors. For instance, one of Brian's clients shared during her first visit that she desired to lose weight but was concerned that she would have a difficult time doing so because of her personal history involving her relationship with and subsequent loss of her mother. This particular client, Robin, told Brian that she felt the most connected and nurtured by her mother when they spent time together baking and eating cookies. Other than these times in the kitchen with her mother, she indicated that she didn't receive much attention or have much of a relationship with her. Whenever life became challenging and overwhelming, whenever feeling lonely, and feeling the need to fill an empty space inside with something, she would consume cookies in large quantities. Through the course of her treatment it became important to find other, healthier ways to fill the void and, through a process of forgiveness, realize the importance of making amends with her mother; otherwise, she would continue to engage in the same behavior pattern that brought her to Brian's office.

When working with obese individuals, it is important to sensitively explore their personal stories for histories of physical and/or sexual abuse. Many, though by no means all, obese individuals struggling with weight management have traumatic histories involving sexual or physical abuse at some time in their lives. Excessive weight at some point in time became a literal and symbolic way for them to maintain a protective barrier from further abuse. Being obese, though perhaps not consciously preferred, offers a sense of safety and security. After all, as one of David's clients frequently voiced, "Who would want to be with someone as fat as me?"

By the same token, excessive weight may be perceived (real or imagined) by the person as a function of strength. It gives them a sense of being more solid, allowing them to (literally) "throw their weight around" to maintain a barrier against sexuality and intimacy. When sexuality and intimacy have been associated with abuse, pain, anger, and hate, much therapeutic work is needed to undo the harmful associations that have been solidified in the person's dysfunctional history. Like Pavlov's dogs, conditioned to salivate to the sound of a bell, a process of extinction will be necessary for the person to be able to feel more comfortable with intimacy. Unfortunately, over time, this unhealthy association fostered a pattern of approach-avoidance fueled by fear and lack of trust that is necessary for intimacy.

It has been our experience that some women (more so than men) who have unsatisfying marriages may gain weight or fail to lose excessive weight as a means of fending off unwanted desires to engage in extramarital affairs. Because this kind of behavior is incongruent with their values and morals, excessive weight solidifies their resistance to the urge, minimizing the risk that they will behave in ways that will ultimately be regretted.

Personal histories may also expose an individual's fear of changing, particularly if the change involves weight loss. For these individuals, there is a risk to losing weight that they may not want to tempt to fate: rejection, lack of support, or jealousy of family members. In many cases, obesity is a family problem; consequently, as one family member becomes permanently fit and trim, others may become resentful, angry, jealous, and may even reject the now thinner person. Addressing these dynamics in ways mentioned above and throughout this book can minimize any undue influence of a sabotaging family member. At times, we have found it beneficial to involve other family members in treatment, whether to solidify support of our client or provide assistance to the client's significant others who may also desire a more fit and healthy body.

THE FAB FOUR

We have identified what we believe to be four very powerful, though frequently overlooked, reasons to change: modeling, personal mastery, freedom, and spirituality. As mentioned above, we want to elicit these reasons from our clients and not simply "feed" them these ideas. Doing so allows them to take ownership of these reasons, which in turn enhances motivation and facilitates greater internal locus of control.

Steve Garvey, the Los Angeles Dodgers' first baseman Hall of Famer, was David's childhood hero. In his mind, Steve Garvey could do no wrong. When playing baseball, whether through an organized league or backyard whiffle ball, David emulated Steve Garvey in every imaginable way possible—the way he threw a ball, maintained a batting stance, or walked on and off the field. Though not much thicker than the handle of his baseball bat, David imagined his forearms to be the Popeye-sized arms sported by his hero. Personal models, be they childhood heroes or current inspirations, offer all of us the opportunity to grow (or unfortunately, in some cases, decompensate) emotionally, behaviorally, and spiritually. Helping our clients identify with someone they admire, whether it is for the body they maintain or for their persistence, drive, ambition, or accomplishments, can provide the additional motivation needed to stay focused on their goal.

For this reason, we generally ask our clients to identify people they respect and admire who can serve as an inspiration to remain committed to their life goals. These people can be personally familiar to your client or, as Steve Garvey was for David, they can be known only through the media or historical records. Some of our clients have found it very beneficial to have pictures of these people near and around them. And because humans tend to be creatures of habit, we encourage them to change the pictures from time to time so they don't become part of the household furniture and lose the inspirational pull they once had.

By the same token, we believe it can be helpful for people to recognize how they serve as role models for others, especially young children if they are involved in their lives. Empirical studies have shown that parents are very influential on children's lifestyle when it comes to fitness and smoking. Families who value fitness and health, either by directly engaging in physical activities with their children, modeling healthy behaviors, or supporting fitness-based activities, significantly reduce the risk of obesity (Anderssen & Wold, 1992; Stucky-Ropp & DiLorenzo, 1993; Trost et al., 2003).

Likewise, when it comes to cigarette smoking, parental smoking cessation has been associated with less adolescent smoking, except when the other parent continued to smoke (Chassin, Presson, Rose, Sherman, & Prost, 2002). And children of smokers are more likely to smoke and maintain more favorable attitudes toward smoking than children of nonsmokers (Andersen, Leroux, Bricker, Rajan, & Peterson, 2004; Wilkinson, Shete, & Prokhorov, 2008).

Personal mastery tends to be overlooked by clients when it comes to habit control; however, we maintain that it is important to elicit this from our clients to help promote desired change of unwanted behaviors. When musicians, martial artists, or athletes experience a sense of personal mastery and behavioral control, they tend to be internally motivated and energized in ways that promote behavioral change. Usually people tend to build upon elementary skills once they experience personal mastery over something.

By the same token, gaining a sense of freedom from addiction, compulsion, or dependence is not only liberating, but reinforces the notion that one can gain a greater sense of control over one's life and behavior than one may have believed. By strategically offering interventions that one our clients elicit a sense of freedom from the destructive behaviors that have in many ways consumed their existence, we afford them a perspective of themselves that may have never before been fully appreciated.

Finally, we believe it is beneficial if not critical to elicit a sense of spirituality by gaining greater control over and respect and appreciation for their bodies, which for years have been abused or at the very least taken for granted. As you may have already surmised, this sense of spirituality ties in with gaining and fostering a greater sense of freedom from addiction, compulsion, or dependence, whether with respect to food, nicotine, alcohol, or drugs.

Ultimately, our goal in eliciting these reasons is to help our clients create a powerful sense of purpose. After all, purpose drives motivation. By eliciting the reasons in a comprehensive manner, we believe you will create a level of motivation that exceeds that which would be expected from an individual who identifies only "improved health" or "saving money" as the primary reason for eliminating unwanted habits in his life.

We want to capitalize on their sense of physical, mental, and emotional growth and development. We want our clients to appreciate the personal, social, and environmental benefits to breaking their habits. To make our efforts more comprehensive in nature, we incorporate their present and their future and do so through hypnotic interventions that rely upon guided imagery and accessing and mobilizing subconscious resources that minimize discomfort while enhancing motivation to achieve their goal of habit control.

ACCESSING AND MOBILIZING RESOURCES

The interventions utilized in this text offer clients alternative ways to satisfy their personal intentions while managing overwhelming stress that leads to smoking and overeating and deflates one's motivation for exercising.

One seemingly simple message that we give to our clients echoes the famous Nike slogan, "Just do it." Brian likes to share a personal rule with his clients that goes like this: "Don't fine-tune what you are not doing." People spend more time preparing to initiate an exercise regimen only to never get it going. Whether they join local gyms, purchase exercise equipment, or engage in hours of research seeking the best running shoe they can buy, in the end, after all is said and done, they still find themselves sitting on the couch watching television or sitting in front of a computer screen or video game. The best preparation in the world, including determining how, when, and where someone should exercise, will never do the necessary work for a person. For people who are trying to determine how they can get the maximum gain from their exercise regimen, or if they should exercise at 70% of their maximum heart rate for 20 or 30 minutes, we tell them that all that doesn't really matter if they aren't *doing* anything. After all, one cannot fine-tune that which is not being done. As renowned Jedi Master Yoda said, "Do...or do not. There is no *try*."

As an avid runner, David understands well how readily he can talk himself out of going for a run in subfreezing temperatures. Maintaining the "Just Do It" philosophy, he will at least lace up his shoes, head out the door, put one foot in front of the other and see where it leads him. Some days, it may be a walk through the neighborhood or a slow jog around the block a few times. Some days, even when the body seems less than willing, the effort pays off and turns into a 6-mile run capped off by a few minutes of jumping rope.

Understanding that all of us have likely had some experience in life in which we applied the "Just Do It" philosophy, whether it was exercising, doing homework, going to work, or starting on some seemingly overwhelming project, we help our clients tap into these successful experiences in an effort to promote the level of motivation needed to just get going. In essence, we consider the past to be a repository of wisdom and experience that we help our clients access.

Milton Erickson was a master when it came to helping people access and mobilize resources that moved them into a healthier emotional, physical, and spiritual future. In fact, Erickson gained an appreciation of the mind's healing capacity when, at the age of 17, he was stricken with polio and overnight was changed from an athlete into a young man critically near death's door. His physician informed his mother that he would probably not live through the night; however, being a strong-willed individual, he vowed that he would not die without seeing one more sunset. So he requested that his mother reposition the dresser with an attached mirror so that he could have a clearer view of the west window of the house. He was able to see the sunset, then collapsed into unconsciousness for 3 days. When he awoke, he asked his family where the fence, boulder, and tree were. They had no clue what he was talking about, thinking he was delirious. Erickson, however, realized these were the last things he saw in his mind before losing consciousness. Years later, he understood that what he had experienced was an altered state of consciousness.

A long, tedious process of recuperation followed the onset of his illness. Due to the crippling effects of the polio, Erickson was confined to his bedroom most of the day while his family worked the farmland outside. Knowing he wanted to be close to his family, they placed him by a window, in a rocking chair with a hole in the seat, beneath which was placed a potty. Thanks in part to his family's oversight one day in forgetting to move his chair to the window, Erickson fortuitously became his own healer. Intently focused on recalling what it felt like to put pressure on the arms of the chair, press his feet on the floorboard, lift himself out of the chair and step with one foot then the other, with his eyes closed, Erickson held these mental images in mind, recalling each muscular movement as precisely as his memory would permit. Within time, he had moved his chair to the window, where he was able to observe his family in the yard below. Over a period of several weeks, through this internal visualization process, he regained the use of his muscles and relearned how to walk (Rosen, 1982). Shortly thereafter, he embarked on a solitary 10-week canoe trip down the Wisconsin River from Milwaukee to St. Louis on the Mississippi, and then paddling back upstream to Milwaukee. When he left, he walked with the assistance of crutches. When he returned, he brought back a wealth of knowledge and the strength to ditch his crutches, replacing them with a cane.

It is via this process of visualization through our hypnotic work that we enable our clients to initiate the changes they seek for themselves, by offering them the opportunity to set the stage for these changes. We help them identify particular resources that they believe they need, such as enhanced attention and concentration, courage, or the capacity to make good choices to succeed. Relying on models to help them through this process, we ask them to identify someone they know, be it a personal friend, public figure, historical figure, or celebrity who can do that which they wish to be able to do. Through trance, we work through a number of steps to help elicit the resource they believe they need.

First, we suggest they imagine seeing and hearing their identified person engage in activities that depict the resource the client desires. They may imagine the model making good choices at a buffet, behaving in a confident manner, remaining calm and in control, exercising, or behaving in ways that are conducive to reaching the identified goal.

Then we encourage our client to imagine his or her model exhibiting these resources in the client's situation and context, but have him or her do it with the client's face and body. So, in essence, it is the model's behavior within the client's body.

Next we suggest the client add the feelings, attitudes, and behaviors to her own personality, her own style, own touch, her own adjustment of this resource. So, at this point in time, it is the client seeing and hearing herself exhibiting this resource in her own way and in her own situation.

Finally, we have the client imagine that he can effortlessly float into the picture. Now we tell the client that he can see himself through his own eyes, hear through his own ears, and feel in his own body this resource that he is experiencing and exhibiting. We further encourage the client to embellish and elaborate on the experience so that it becomes his alone. Again, this is a process of eliciting internal resources while facilitating an internal locus of control for the client so it can become part of his personal history.

CUES AND TRIGGERS

As we help clients elicit, access, and mobilize resources, we can begin to explore the cues and triggers that precipitate unwanted habit behavior. We identify and address three general categories of cues and triggers with our clients, including people, places, and activities.

People tend to be a primary cue for smokers to light up a cigarette and also serve as triggers that lead to relapse. Exploring a client's smoking history can be important for determining the influence that other people have on their smoking behavior. Some people are very concerned about feeling left out of a group, so they continue to smoke socially. They may also feel a certain kind of peer pressure to smoke, and this is a particularly troublesome issue for teenagers and young adults. People are also a source of stress for others and consequently this stressor triggers individuals to continue to smoke. As we mentioned earlier, parents who smoke tend to influence their children, who are at greater risk for becoming smokers than children living with nonsmoking parents.

Interventions to address people's triggers for smoking include: temporarily breaking off relations with other smokers, if possible; going to nonsmoking establishments; and learning more effective and healthy ways to manage stress associated with certain relationships.

Individuals who overeat also identify people as triggers or cues for overeating. Again, stressors associated with people are likely to be embedded in their personal history and can be a recurring source of conflict and stress that promotes overeating. Families who tend to eat unhealthy meals, visit fast-food restaurants, or simply fail to endorse a healthy lifestyle may trigger unhealthy eating habits. It all begins at the grocery store; consequently, if your client lives in a home where someone else does the shopping, it will be important for your client to gain greater control over the food that is brought into the home. Otherwise, if, like most of us, the client tends to eat what is available, he and his body are at the mercy of the household's designated shopper.

It is difficult to simply avoid other family members when it comes to establishing a healthier lifestyle and diet; however, people can be empowered to take charge of their own well-being, direct their own grocery shopping, and perhaps influence others in the home to join them in their quest to become permanently fit and trim.

Certain places, usually because of repeated associations with smoking or stress eating, can also serve as triggers and cues to maintain unhealthy habits. Bars and restaurants notoriously serve as triggers for people to overeat, smoke, and consume alcoholic beverages. For some people, it may be their kitchen or living room, a screened-in porch, or in front of a computer. One of David's clients reported that 80% of his smoking was done while working on his computer. He kept an ashtray within reach, right next to his lighter and pack of cigarettes. To help break this chain of behaviors, David encouraged him to keep his cigarettes and his lighter in more inconvenient places and separate from each other, like the top of a cupboard or bookshelf. Each time a cigarette was desired, the client had to leave his computer, walk across the room, reach for his pack of cigarettes, retrieve a cigarette, then walk to the opposite side of the room and retrieve his lighter. Obviously, this plan takes a sense of will and determination to follow through with the imposed suggestion. In this particular case, this and other interventions (e.g., hypnosis, EFT, nicotine gum) have been helpful in allowing David's client to stop smoking.

By identifying a pattern of behavior and paying particular attention to the environment, we can establish interventions that break the routines that maintain the unwanted habit. We have found it particularly helpful to have our clients write down a detailed sequence of events that leads to the unwanted habit. We then review the sequence, searching for ways to disrupt or alter it in some ways that facilitate a change in behavior. For some of our smoking clients, we encourage them to smoke with the opposite hand; and if they consume coffee with their cigarette, we may have them prepare their coffee in a slightly different way (less sugar, more cream, or black) and also drink it using the opposite hand. For clients who smoke inside their home, we encourage them to smoke outside. This is usually a welcome change for any nonsmokers in the house, who appreciate the efforts, which ultimately serve as reinforcement for our client.

PUTTING IT INTO ACTION

After eliciting from a client the reasons to change, the reasons for becoming a permanent nonsmoker or for becoming permanently fit and trim, we introduce them to a metaphor that puts decision making into a slightly different context for them. For many people, the choice to smoke or the choice to eat something unhealthy is set up and perceived by them in ways that make smoking a cigarette or eating a piece of cake inviting, if not compelling. For them, the choice appears to be between smoking and not smoking or between eating a piece of cake and not eating a piece of cake.

We tell our clients that these aren't really the choices before them. To make this more pragmatic, we suggest that they imagine being involved in a game show. And in this game show they have a choice of the prize behind Door #1 (we point to the right, or the client's left and a bit behind them) or Door #2 (we then point to the left, or just in front of the client's right side). We tell them that behind Door #1 are all the cigarettes they could smoke or all the cheesecake they could eat. We discuss all of the things behind Door #1 as if it were in their past, a way they had once dealt with stress. We might say, "And behind that door are all the cigarettes you could smoke. Those are the cigarettes that may have helped you deal with stress, or cope with difficult times you've had in your life."

Behind Door #2, again pointing toward their right, just in front of them, we tell them, is "an improved quality of life, improved health and freedom from disease, being a model of health and good judgment for others, having more energy and vitality, and being able to comfortably engage in activities, doing this with and for the ones you love. Behind this door is the opportunity to have more money, to have greater control over your destiny, and to live life with the values you hold to be true."

After making these options clear to them, we then ask them to select a door. Pointing back toward Door #2 we remind them that selecting Door #2 tells us that the choice is not just between a cigarette and not a cigarette or a piece of cake and not a piece of cake. We then pull out the piece of paper with the list of all the reasons they identified for choosing to become permanent nonsmokers or permanently fit and trim. Reading off the reasons to them helps them make a more conscious decision about smoking or choosing unhealthy foods to consume.

This process sets up our next intervention, which involves effectively setting and reaching well-formed goals and desired outcomes. In the next chapter, we review ways to help clients attain their goals through creating a new self-image that is inviting, compelling, and magnetic.

CONCLUSION

In this chapter, we discussed the importance of helping our clients identify reasons for changing unwanted habits by having them consider the benefits of improved appearance, logistics, financial benefits, and enhanced physical and mental abilities. We also identified four primary areas to consider when eliciting change from our clients (emotional, physical, logistical, and personal) in addition to four very powerful, though frequently overlooked reasons to change (modeling, personal mastery, freedom, and spirituality).

Knowing change can be difficult to initiate and maintain, we employ visualization techniques with our clients, knowing that these techniques can foster motivation, drive, and persistence. First, we suggest they imagine seeing and hearing an identified role model engage in activities that depict the resource the client desires. Then we encourage them to imagine their model exhibiting these resources in the client's situation, context, and body. Next we suggest the client add the feelings, attitudes, and behaviors to their own personality, their own style, their own touch, their own use of this resource. Finally, we tell the clients to see themselves through their own eyes, hear through their own ears, and feel in their own bodies this resource that they are experiencing and exhibiting. We further encourage them to embellish and elaborate on the experience so that it becomes personalized.

As we help clients elicit, access, and mobilize resources, it is also important to identify the cues and triggers that precipitate unwanted habit behavior. Doing so allows for an essential relapse-prevention plan. Examining cues and triggers and heading them off as soon as possible greatly reduces risk of relapse while promoting permanent habit control.

Things to Do

1. Identify with your client or yourself positive reasons (emotional, physical, logistical, and personal) for changing or maintaining unwanted behavior.
2. Identify cues and triggers that maintain the unwanted behavior and strategies to minimize the unwanted behavior from ever re-occurring.
3. Practice guided-imagery techniques, suggested above, and record yourself so that you can review the recording and identify ways to enhance your performance. You may learn that you talk too slowly, too fast, too loudly, too softly, and so on, and will be able to make appropriate adjustments.

5

Knowledge Is Power:
The Skinny on the Fat and
Clearing the Smoke in the Air

All truths are easy to understand once they are discovered; the point is to discover them.

—Galileo Galilei

When working with clients seeking assistance with weight management, smoking cessation, or some other health-related concern, we as providers are obligated to remain informed about the latest research and contemporary developments in the health care field. At the same time, we must maintain an acute awareness of the misinformation that is perpetuated by the mass media and be prepared to educate our clients and provide them with accurate information, particularly if it is relevant to their treatment. Possessing a working knowledge of experimental design and statistical analysis will permit a more critical analysis of purported research results. Though it is not necessary to be able to calculate an analysis of variance, one should be able to understand the difference between a controlled and uncontrolled study and between one that has random assignment of subjects to experimental and controll groups and a study that includes preselected subjects.

To illustrate this point, by now we are all aware of the general consensus put forth in the media, and now indicated as a black box warning, that selective serotonin reuptake inhibitors (SSRIs) are associated with an increased risk of suicidality in children and adolescents. Controlled studies, however, have generally indicated that the benefits of medication for the treatment of depression and anxiety in children and adolescents far outweigh the risks of suicidal thoughts or behavior (Bridge et al., 2007). In fact, when cautious reports were first put forth, a number of extraneous variables were neglected in the final analysis that led to the conclusions that SSRI medication was contraindicated in children. Such factors as subclinical medication dosing by primary care physicians and pediatricians, poor compliance with medication regimens, failure to appropriately increase and/or titrate medication, and misdiagnosis were generally not considered influential variables in the increased risk of suicidality for adolescents prescribed an SSRI. Rather, if the child displayed suicidality and had been taking (or prescribed) an SSRI, the correlation alone was assumed to be causative; hence the alarming concern on behalf of the Food and Drug Administration and the mass media, which expediently shared this information with the general public.

MATCHING INFORMATION

We previously emphasized the importance of assessment and establishing rapport in gaining a better understanding of our clients as we work with them and help address their unwanted habits. In chapter 4, we reviewed ways to solicit reasons for changing, ensuring that the client has consciously considered change so that she becomes empowered to establish and seek an identified goal. Further, this information provides us with personal information to facilitate an individualized treatment plan.

In an effort to facilitate greater levels of motivation for fostering change, we believe it is vital to provide our clients with accurate information. Some clients are information junkies and actively seek whatever information they can find to enhance their knowledge base. They are the people who know every ball player's batting average, every pitcher's earned run average, every quarterback's pass-rating score. Others have little use for information and just want the bottom-line facts or general information that they can use.

Some people prefer an overview or the "Cliff's Notes" version and have no desire to know specific details. Others want the details only after they have been given an overview. As we discussed in chapter 3 (on the Enneagram), there is a personality type, called The Investigator, who spends time and energy gathering information.

When determining what and how much information to provide to our clients, we consider information that moves an individual *toward* motivation as well as information that moves an individual *away from* motivation. The former involves empowerment, whereas the latter is fear-based. Both can be effective, though, for some, fear-based information works best, whereas for others knowledge that empowers is most effective. When providing clients with information that is fear-based, care must be taken to ensure that the data supplied doesn't upset them to such an extent that they avoid information altogether and thereby enhance the likelihood that the unwanted behavior will persist. For instance, there is the old joke about the smoker who, after reading the warning labels on cigarette packs, became so upset that he decided to stop reading. By the same token, enhanced anxiety or fear can be helpful if, for instance, someone fails to use their seatbelt until they see a picture of a traumatic accident scene involving an unrestrained passenger.

It is also important to consider the client's values that were shared during the initial assessment meetings. This information can be used in ways that allow us to offer information to a client that is couched in terms that fit well with the client's personal values. Biblical references about health, for instance, wouldn't be particularly helpful to a secularist agnostic or atheist, but it may be very beneficial to a born-again Christian.

A client's knowledge base, as discussed previously, should be considered when providing relevant information or clinical research. It has been our experience that when it comes to weight loss, clients frequently come in with a plethora of information. It is likely that they have read several diet and nutrition books, been to Weight Watchers and Jenny Craig, and know all they need to know about counting calories and carbohydrates.

And if some clients come to your office armed with notebooks full of information, one cannot assume that all of it is good, accurate, or relevant. At times, it is incumbent upon the therapist to validate the information by accessing reputable sources of data and information or at the very least guiding our clients to these sources.

Knowing a client's academic history, vocabulary, and reading interests can help guide the process for sharing information with her. We can then determine the amount of material and specific details that would or would not be beneficial for the client. Discussing the caloric index of foods or body mass index calculations may not be necessary for clients who simply need to be told what kind of food to avoid and what kind of food would be healthier to consume.

BEHIND THE SMOKE SCREEN

Most people are cognizant of the four primary health-related illnesses associated with smoking: lung cancer, emphysema, heart disease, and cerebrovascular accidents. Throughout the body every cell that requires oxygen and every cell that relies on nutrition from blood and the lymphatic system is adversely impacted by smoking. Unbeknownst to many, smokers have twice the rate of back pain as nonsmokers. In recent years, researchers have uncovered a surprising connection between smoking and back pain. The trend holds for men and women, for manual laborers and white-collar workers alike. The investigations raise interesting questions about the root causes of pain and, on a more practical level, give smokers a whole new reason to quit.

A study published in the *Annals of the Rheumatic Diseases* (Palmer, Syddall, Cooper, & Coggon, 2003) drives the point home. British researchers asked nearly 13,000 people about their lifestyles, including their smoking habits, jobs, activity levels, and history of pain. After adjusting for the demands of strenuous jobs and other factors that might cause back pain, the scientists concluded that smoking—by itself—raised the risk of debilitating back pain by about 30%. Smoking also seemed to make people slightly more vulnerable to pain in the neck, shoulders, elbows, hands, hips, and knees. Further, the authors concluded that regional pain was also greater for ex-smokers than those who never smoked.

Their report is not alone in its conclusions. An article recently published in *Spine* by Mikkonen and colleagues (2008) concluded that "regular smoking in adolescence was associated with low back pain in young adults."

Scientists aren't sure why some smokers are prone to back pain. According to the aforementioned report in the *Annals of the Rheumatic Diseases* (Palmer et al., 2003), nicotine from cigarettes "could affect the manner in which the brain processes sensory stimuli and the central perception of pain." In other words, cigarettes affect the way the brain sends its pain signals. Smoking may also damage tissue in the lower back and elsewhere in the body by slowing down circulation and reducing the flow of nutrients to joints and muscles.

Cigarette smoke is well recognized as an immunosuppressant. More specifically, in their comprehensive review of smoking and its immunosuppressant properties, Mehta, Nazzal, and Sadikot (2008) note how smoking affects host innate immunity, including structural and functional changes in the respiratory ciliary epithelium, lung surfactant protein, and immune cells such as alveolar macrophages, neutrophils, lymphocytes, and natural killer cells. Additionally, there is preliminary, though not conclusive, evidence that smoking is directly related to disorders that affect vision, including cataracts and macular degeneration (see Lois et al., 2008).

According to the Centers for Disease Control and Prevention (CDC), approximately 440,000 people in the United States died in 2004 from tobacco use. Nearly one of every five deaths was related to smoking, and cigarettes kill more Americans than alcohol, car accidents, suicide, homicide, and illegal drug use combined. The American Cancer Society (ACS) has claimed that in 2002 cancer overtook heart disease as the number one cause of death in Americans under age 85; however, this statistic has not held up over time. Nonetheless, the ACS maintains that one-third of all cancer deaths are due to smoking and another third are due to obesity and poor diet. Obesity comes in a close second as killer of people and in the near future may surpass cigarette smoking as the number one cause of preventable death.

There are two health issues that we find particularly motivating and compelling for people: wrinkles and erectile dysfunction (ED). Long-term smoking produces detrimental effects on the vascular endothelium and peripheral nerves and also causes ultrastructural damage to the corporal tissue, all of which are considered to play a significant role in chronic smoking-induced ED, risk of ED, or a history of ED (Tostes et al., 2008). This information may be helpful for reinforcing an individual's desire for and dedication to becoming a permanent nonsmoker. It has been our experience in our own practices that some male smokers complaining of ED were unaware that smoking contributes to this most troubling disorder. Thus, it may behoove you to inquire about ED during your initial interview with your male clients.

There is ample evidence linking smoking and dermatological changes, including premature skin aging, poor wound healing, squamous cell carcinoma, melanoma, oral cancer, acne, psoriasis, and hair loss (Morita, 2007). Unfortunately, though young women smokers in particular identify concerns about the effects of smoking on physical appearance, especially yellowed teeth and wrinkled skin, they are not likely to quit smoking until the negative effects on appearance become noticeable, by which time issues such as dependence and engrained habit make quitting more challenging (Grogan, Fry, Gough, & Conner, 2009).

Whereas most informed people understand that smoking is a tremendous health risk, very few could tell you the process by which these health risks occur. In an effort to explain the process in terms that are easily explained and understood, we use the following metaphor, which we find helpful: Oxygen, hemoglobin, and the locomotive. We tell our clients that hemoglobin, which is a part of our red blood cells, transports oxygen from our lungs to every cell in the body. Unfortunately, hemoglobin also has a stronger affinity or attraction to carbon monoxide than to oxygen. Consequently, many of our red blood cells will carry carbon monoxide rather than oxygen if we have been exposed to carbon monoxide (automobile exhaust, cigarette smoke, furnaces, gas heaters, fireplaces).

Using the analogy of an old-style locomotive train we tell our patients to consider that their body is like a locomotive and that it needs coal (oxygen-rich hemoglobin) to move. We then ask our clients to consider what would happen if the firebox on a locomotive were smaller than it should be and half of the coal used to propel the train didn't burn and the train was traveling uphill. Surely, they conclude, the train will move slowly and may not make it up the hill. We then tell them that carbon monoxide from cigarette smoke restricts the amount of oxygen in the hemoglobin and also constricts blood vessels (much as the smaller firebox promotes inefficient coal burning). Consequently, if only half of the coal shoveled into the firebox is burning and the opening of the firebox is much smaller, the train is going to huff-puff just like any winded, oxygen-deprived smoker taking a brisk walk.

At times we encounter the naysayer who espouses a "What does it matter?" attitude, believing he is going to be ill anyway or think it's too late to quit now. It is therefore very important to let clients know how well the body rejuvenates once smoking ceases. The informative

Table 5.1

PHYSICAL CHANGES AFTER THE LAST CIGARETTE*

AFTER SMOKING THAT LAST CIGARETTE

20 Minutes After Quitting: Your heart rate drops.

12 Hours After Quitting: Carbon monoxide level in your blood drops to normal.

2 Weeks to 3 Months After Quitting: Your heart attack risk begins to drop. Your lung function begins to improve.

1 to 9 Months After Quitting: Your coughing and shortness of breath decrease.

1 Year After Quitting: Your added risk of coronary heart disease is half that of a smoker's.

5 Years After Quitting: Your stroke risk is reduced to that of a nonsmoker's 5 to 15 years after quitting.

10 Years After Quitting: Your lung cancer death rate is about half that of a smoker's. Your risk of cancers of the mouth, throat, esophagus, bladder, kidney, and pancreas decreases.

15 Years After Quitting: Your risk of coronary heart disease is back to that of a nonsmoker's.

*From National Center for Chronic Disease Prevention and Health Promotion.

chart above (Table 5.1), from the National Center for Chronic Disease Prevention and Health Promotion, includes two elements of educational information we encourage you to copy and provide to your client.

The upper portion reviews the changes that occur within the body within a specified time after an individual smokes that last cigarette. For instance, 20 minutes after smoking a cigarette, a smoker's heart rate drops; 1 year after quitting, the risk of coronary disease is half that of a smoker; and 15 years after quitting, the risk of coronary disease returns to that of a nonsmoker.

The lower portion of the table reviews the improved health and reduced illness and disease risks associated with quitting smoking. For example, bladder cancer and peripheral artery disease are reduced significantly just a few years after quitting smoking.

THE SKINNY ON THE FAT

The Body Mass Index (BMI) is a screening tool used to measure weight relative to height. Although BMI does not measure body fat directly, it has been shown to correlate with measures of body fat, such as underwater weighing, and is considered an accurate alternative for body fat measurement. To calculate your BMI, you will need to divide your weight in pounds by your height in inches squared and multiply that by 703. The formula for calculating BMI is:

$$\text{Weight} / [\text{Height (in inches)}]^2 \times 703$$

The CDC Web page offers separate, easy-to-use BMI calculators for adults and for children and adolescents that can be accessed at the following link:

http://www.cdc.gov/nccdphp/dnpa/healthyweight/assessing/bmi/index.htm

Scores below 18.5 are considered underweight; scores between 18.5 and 24.9 are within the normal weight range; scores between 25.0 to 29.9 are classified as overweight; and scores 30 and above are classified as obese. Referring back to the shaded map of the United States in chapter 1, we can see how obesity has been on the rise and continues to climb with each decade that passes.

It is important to remember, however, that BMI is not a direct measure of "body fatness" and that BMI is calculated from an individual's weight, which includes both muscle and fat. Consequently, some individuals may have a high BMI but not have a high percentage of body fat. For example, highly trained athletes may have a high BMI because of increased muscularity rather than increased body fatness. Although some people with a BMI in the overweight range (25.0–29.9) may not have excess body fatness, most people with a BMI in the obese range (equal to or greater than 30) will have increased levels of body fatness; therefore it is important to consider an individual's body structure when evaluating the calculated BMI figure.

Although BMI is calculated the same way for children and adults, the criteria used to interpret the meaning of the BMI number for children and adolescents are different from those used for adults. For children and teens, BMI age- and gender-specific percentiles are used for two reasons:

- The percentage of body fat changes with age.
- The percentage of body fat differs between girls and boys.

Because of these factors, the interpretation of BMI is both age- and gender-specific for children and teens. The CDC BMI-for-age growth charts take into account these differences and allow for a translation of a BMI number into a percentile for a child's gender and age. For adults, on the other hand, BMI is interpreted through categories that are not dependent on gender or age.

In 1998, the National Heart, Lung, and Blood Institute, a division of the National Institutes of Health, published a comprehensive report detailing clinical findings revealing that as weight increases to reach the levels referred to as "overweight" and "obese," the risk for the following conditions also increases:

- Coronary heart disease
- Type 2 diabetes
- Cancers (endometrial, breast, and colon)
- Hypertension (high blood pressure)
- Dyslipidemia (for example, high total cholesterol or high levels of triglycerides)
- Stroke
- Liver and gallbladder disease
- Sleep apnea and respiratory problems
- Osteoarthritis (a degeneration of cartilage and its underlying bone within a joint)
- Gynecological problems (abnormal menses, infertility)

Fat as a Chemical Factory

It is well established that muscle tissue drives metabolism and greater levels of muscle volume are associated with a higher rate of metabolism. Two men weighing the same, but with different amounts of lean muscle mass, can have very different basal metabolic rates (the minimal caloric requirement needed to sustain life in a resting individual). In other words, basal metabolic rate (BMR) is the number of calories you'd burn if you slept all day. Therefore, while sleeping, an individual with greater muscle mass will have higher levels of metabolic activity than his fatter counterpart. You can find a BMR calculator at the following site: http:// www.consumerstyle.com/calculators/bmr.php.

It has long been proposed by those supposedly in the know that for every pound of new muscle gained, your body will burn an extra 60 calories per day. Unfortunately, this theory just hasn't stood the test of time or scrutiny of empirical research.

It is, however accurate that when an individual gains muscle, his or her resting metabolic rate does increase. But, the enhanced fuel burning is much less than the 50- to 100-calorie figure we often hear espoused by the so called "health experts." This begs the question: So, where did the 50- to 100-calorie figure actually come from?

Who knows? We're not really sure. We chalk it up to another myth that has been so frequently espoused that its accuracy is no longer questioned, and it likely exists for the same reason that other misconceptions remain unchallenged. Somebody says something, somebody repeats it, and then we repeat it. Suddenly it's established as fact. With the advent of the Internet, and e-mail in particular, the exponential growth of urban legends has given birth to an entire Web site dedicated to separating fact from fiction (www.snopes.com).

In studies that have tracked changes in muscle mass and metabolism, it is easy to understand how it appears that the metabolic rate of muscle is somewhere in the region of 50 to 100 calories per pound. But, upon closer inspection, we see that things are not quite so simple and straightforward. Let's look at a few examples.

The first comes from an 18-week study published in the *Journal of Applied Physiology* (Van Etten, Westerterp, Verstappen, Boon, & Saris, 1997) involving 26 sedentary men. During the first 8 weeks, the men gained roughly 2.8 pounds of fat-free muscle mass. Their average daily metabolic rate increased by 263 calories per day. Dividing the increase in resting metabolic rate (263 calories) by the increase in fat-free mass (2.8 pounds) gives us a figure of 94 calories per pound. However, can we really assume that this figure represents the metabolic rate of muscle?

Not quite. The first problem is the daily metabolic rate figure includes the energy cost of physical activity. We can't conclusively conclude that the increase in calorie expenditure was exclusively due to extra muscle growth.

Furthermore, from week 8 to week 18, the men gained another 1.8 pounds of fat-free mass. If muscle had such a big impact on metabolism, we'd expect to see an additional rise in the men's metabolic rate. But that's not what happened. Consequently, we cannot apply a simple formula espousing that adding a pound of muscle mass will burn an additional 50 to 60 calories per day.

In a related study, women who engaged in resistance training 3 days a week for 6 months gained 2.9 pounds of fat-free mass (Poehlman et al., 2002). In that time, their resting metabolic rate increased by an average of 60 calories per day. Dividing the increase in resting metabolic rate (60 calories) by the increase in fat-free mass (2.9 pounds) gives us a figure of 20.7 calories per pound. However, for reasons noted above, this figure overestimates the metabolic rate of muscle.

Methods for measuring resting metabolic rate and body composition vary widely in their precision and accuracy. We cannot be certain if the change in resting metabolism was due to extra muscle mass or to measurement error. The control group in this study did not exercise, yet their resting metabolic rate increased by 31 calories per day.

Other studies have revealed similar findings, revealing increases in resting metabolic rate even when controlling for gains in fat-free mass (Pratley et al., 1994). It is therefore likely that variables other than the increase in fat-free mass (e.g., changes in the activity of the sympathetic nervous system) are partly responsible.

In many people's minds, fat seems to be nothing more than a blob of inert matter. Perhaps as a child you've been told by a critical parent, "Don't just lie there like a lump of fat, get off your butt." But contrary to what many believe, fat is not simply "dead" tissue. It secretes proteins such as leptin and cytokines, which can affect your metabolism (Wajchenberg, 2000). According to some estimates, fat has a daily metabolic rate of 2 calories per pound per day, with muscle clocking in at just 6 calories per pound (Wang, Heshka, Zhang, Boozer, & Heymsfield, 2001).

Fat, we now know, is a potent chemical factory. Unfortunately, it is a very toxic factory that emits all kinds of inflammatory agents affecting several systems throughout our bodies, including the cardio-vascular and hormonal systems.

Fat comes in two main varieties: subcutaneous, which means "under the skin," and visceral, which means "pertaining to the soft organs in the abdomen." Subcutaneous fat is the stuff that jiggles, the fat we hate to see on our bodies. Visceral fat, on the other hand, is not always visible from the outside. It packs itself around the inner organs of the abdomen and sometimes within the liver. Everyone has some visceral fat because it protects our internal organs, acting both as a shock absorber in case of trauma and as an insulator to help us conserve body heat. Visceral fat is actually living, breathing, hormone-producing, metabolically active tissue deep inside our abdominal cavity. It provides storage for energy and rapidly releases energy or fuel into our blood between meals. Visceral fat helps regulate body functions through an active interplay of chemical communications with the central nervous system.

Visceral and adipose tissues make and release a variety of compounds, including enzymes, hormones (e.g., leptin which helps regulate appetite), and inflammation-related chemicals called cytokines. Too much visceral fat leads to a rise in levels of C-reactive protein and other clotting proteins that, when elevated, can cause a metabolic syndrome (high waist size leading to a rise in glucose, high blood pressure, low levels of high-density lipoprotein [HDL, or "good"] cholesterol, and high triglyceride levels).

Although visceral fat and subcutaneous fat are in the same general category, they are quite dissimilar. Apple-shaped bodies compared to pear-shaped bodies, for example, have more visceral fat, which is more metabolically active than subcutaneous fat, posing a greater risk to the body. Visceral fat decreases insulin sensitivity (making diabetes more likely), increases triglyceride levels, decreases levels of HDL cholesterol, creates more inflammation, and raises blood pressure—all of which increase the risk of heart disease. Visceral fat also releases more of its free fatty acids into the blood stream, further increasing the risk of both diabetes and heart disease. The overall effect of excess visceral fat is that it creates a physical environment that is primed for heart disease and stroke, and greatly increases the risk for certain cancers such as breast and endometrial cancer.

Dieting Smarter, Not Harder

There is probably more "expert" information about what you should and should not eat and strategies for losing or even gaining weight than there is on just about any other subject matter. Of course, not all of this information is accurate or beneficial, and some of it has proven to be harmful (remember the Fen-Phen scare?).

Over the course of the past 10 to 15 years, we have witnessed the rise and fall of various fad diets. The low-fat/no-fat program, which was beneficial for some for fostering weight loss, became a no-win plan for those who binged on bags of low-fat cookies with excessive calories, sugar, and talcum powder–type flour that defeated the purpose of losing weight. This led to the notion that carbohydrate, rather than fat, was the weight-gain culprit, which gave birth to the Atkins Diet plan. The Atkins plan, as you may know, involves a diet low in carbohydrates, which helps regulate insulin production and thereby decrease circulating insulin. Less insulin results in less fat storage and fewer food cravings. Though the information available through mass media outlets would have you believe that there is ample data to support this or any other diet, there is limited, and sometimes no, empirical data to support the efficacy of any of these specialized diets.

What we do know is that it is not the amount of fats or carbohydrates consumed that is important. Rather, it is the quality and type of one or the other that makes the most difference. The major kinds of fats in the foods we consume are saturated, polyunsaturated, monounsaturated and trans fatty acids. Saturated fats and trans fats raise blood cholesterol levels, creating a major risk factor for coronary heart disease, including heart attack and stroke. Monounsaturated fats are found in natural foods such as nuts and avocados and are the main component of tea seed oil and olive oil (oleic acid). Canola oil is 57 to 60% monounsaturated fat, olive oil is about 75% monounsaturated fat, and tea seed oil is commonly over 80% monounsaturated fat. Other sources of monounsaturated fat include grape seed oil, ground nut oil, peanut oil, flaxseed oil, sesame oil, sunflower oil, and avocado oil. Generally speaking, monounsaturated and polyunsaturated (including omega-3 and omega-6) fatty acids lower low-density lipoprotein (LDL, or "bad") cholesterol, while possibly raising high-density lipoprotein (HDL, "good") cholesterol levels. Their true ability to raise HDL cholesterol, however, is still under debate.

Polyunsaturated fat can be found mostly in grain products, fish and seafood (herring, salmon, mackerel, halibut), soybeans, and fish oil. Foods like mayonnaise and soft margarine may also be good sources, but nutritional facts can vary by style and brand. Omega-3 fatty acids in fish oil, fish, and seafood, for instance, have been shown to lower the risk of heart attacks through anti-inflammatory mechanisms (Simopoulos, 2002; Zhao et al., 2009). Omega-6 fatty acids in sunflower oil and safflower oil also reduce the risk of cardiovascular disease, but can contribute to allergies and inflammation, which increase the risk for diseases such as irritable bowel syndrome, Crohn's disease, rheumatoid arthritis, and chronic obstructive pulmonary disease (Simopoulos, 2006).

Most omega-6 fatty acids in the diet are consumed from vegetable oils such as linoleic acid (LA; not to be confused with alpha-linolenic acid [ALA], which is found in omega-3 fatty acids, as mentioned below). LA is converted to gamma-linolenic acid (GLA) in the body and then further broken down to arachidonic acid (AA). AA can also be consumed directly from meat, and GLA can be ingested from several plant-based oils, including evening primrose oil, borage oil, and black currant seed oil.

Excess amounts of LA and AA from omega-6 fatty acids are unhealthy because they promote inflammation (Figure 5.1), leading to several of the diseases described above. In contrast, GLA may actually reduce inflammation. Much of the GLA taken as a supplement is converted not to AA, but rather to a substance called dihomogamma-linolenic acid (DGLA). DGLA competes with AA and prevents the negative inflammatory effects that AA would otherwise cause in the body. In addition, DGLA becomes part of a particular series of substances, called prostaglandins, which can reduce inflammation. Having adequate amounts of certain nutrients in the body (including magnesium, zinc, and vitamins C, B3, and B6) helps promote the conversion of GLA to DGLA rather than AA.

Recently, there has been a dramatic surge in interest, among the public and health professionals alike, of the health effects of omega-3 fatty acids derived from fish and fish oils—consisting of docosahexaenoic acid (DHA) plus eicosapentaenoic acid (EPA). DHA is required in high levels in the brain and retina as a physiologically essential nutrient providing for optimal neuronal functioning (learning ability, mental development) and visual acuity, in young and old alike. DHA plus EPA are both considered to have beneficial effects in the prevention and management of cardiovascular disease as well as other chronic disorders, including inflammatory and autoimmune diseases (Simopoulos, 2006). Whereas considerable amounts of ALA are consumed daily in North America (approximately 2 g/day), the physiologically essential nutrient DHA is consumed at lower levels (approximately 80 mg/day). EPA in contrast is consumed at approximately 50 mg/day in a typical North American diet.

Though this may be more information than your client may ever need or desire (and a bit technical at that), we believe it is important to have a basic understanding of what constitutes a healthy diet. We therefore encourage our clients to consume healthy fats while minimizing saturated, hydrogenated, and trans (partially hydrogenated) fats.

The Glycemic Index: All Carbs Are Not Created Equal

Not all carbohydrate foods are created equal. In fact, they behave quite differently in our bodies. The glycemic index (GI) describes this difference by ranking carbohydrates according to their effect on our blood glucose levels. Selecting low-GI carbohydrates—the ones that produce only small fluctuations in our blood glucose and insulin levels—is the secret to long-term cardiovascular benefits and the key to sustainable weight loss.

The GI is a ranking of carbohydrates on a scale from 0 to 100 according to the extent to which they raise blood sugar levels after eating. Foods with a high GI are those which are rapidly digested and absorbed and result in marked fluctuations in blood sugar levels. Low-GI foods, by virtue of their slow digestion and absorption, produce gradual rises in blood sugar and insulin levels and have proven benefits for health. Low-GI diets have been shown to improve both glucose and lipid levels in people with both type 1 and type 2 diabetes. They are particularly beneficial for weight management because they help control appetite and delay hunger. Low-GI diets also reduce insulin levels and insulin resistance.

Recent studies indicate that the risks of diseases such as type 2 diabetes and coronary heart disease are strongly related to the GI of the overall diet (Gutschall, Miller, Mitchell, & Lawrence, 2009; Miller, Gutschall, & Mitchell, 2009). In 1998, the World Health Organization (WHO) and Food and Agriculture Organization (FAO) recommended that people in industrialized countries base their diets on low-GI foods so as to prevent the most common diseases of affluence, such as coronary disease, diabetes, and obesity.

To determine a food's GI rating, measured portions of the food containing 10 to 50 grams of carbohydrate are fed to 10 healthy people

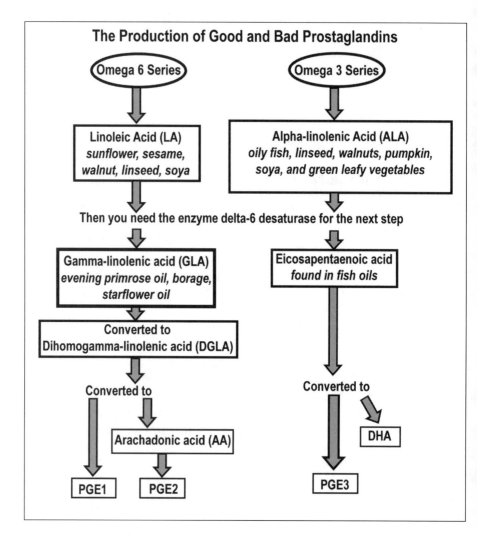

Figure 5.1 Production of good (anti-inflammatory) and bad (inflammatory) prostagladins. Adapted from Glenville (2001).

after an overnight fast. Finger-prick blood samples are taken at 15- to 30-minute intervals over the next 2 hours. These blood samples are used to construct a blood sugar response curve for the 2-hour period. The area under the curve (AUC) is calculated to reflect the total rise in blood glucose levels after eating the test food. The GI rating (%) is calculated by dividing the AUC for the test food by the AUC for the reference food (same amount of glucose) and multiplying by 100. The use of a standard food is essential for reducing the confounding influence of differences in the physical characteristics of the subjects. The average of the GI ratings from all ten subjects is published as the GI of that food.

The GI is the measurement of how different carbohydrates impact blood glucose levels, how high they go up, how fast they go up, and in what way they go up. It is divided into high, medium, and low-GI foods. For instance, a high-GI food like glucose, which is what most of the glycemic indexes are based on, has a score of 100. When you take in glucose, your blood sugar rises very, very quickly and becomes very high.

The glycemic index of foods has significant implications for the food industry. While the Food and Drug Administration in the United States is behind the times with the GI, some foods on the Australian market already show their GI rating on the nutrition information panel. Terms such as complex carbohydrates and sugars, which commonly appear on food labels, are now recognized as having little nutritional or physiological significance. The World Health Organization recommended that these terms be removed and replaced with the total carbohydrate content of the food and its GI value. However, the GI rating of a food must be tested physiologically, and only a few centers around the world currently provide a legitimate testing service. The Human Nutrition Unit at the University of Sydney has been at the forefront of GI research for over two decades and has tested hundreds of foods as an integral part of its program. Jennie Brand Miller is a major contributor to the International Tables of Glycemic Index initially published by the *American Journal of Clinical Nutrition* in 1995 (Foster-Powell & Brand-Miller, 1995) and more recently revised in 2002. (Foster-Powell, Holt, & Brand-Miller, 2002)

Some of the complaints about the glycemic index are that it is too difficult to calculate and that many diverse common foods have similar GI values; for example, melba toast, bagels, white bread, 100% whole wheat bread, angel food cake, graham crackers, whole wheat crackers, couscous, corn chips, oatmeal muffins, french fries, mashed potatoes, canned green pea soup, and the breakfast cereals Cream of Wheat, Cheerios, and Golden Grahams have almost identical GI values (range, 94–106). On the other hand, the GI values of some foods can vary markedly, depending on variety, processing, and preparation. This does not necessarily invalidate the GI concept, but it does make it more difficult to apply in practice than other dietary reference numbers at our disposal. For example, there are many varieties of rice with different types of starch, processed in different ways, that result in different GI values; for example, the GI of 1-inch cubes of boiled potato can be increased by 25% by mashing them, and subtle differences in ripeness can double a banana's glycemic index.

On the other hand, many foods are fairly consistent when tested in different facilities. Though somewhat complicated, given the above variables, motivated individuals may be able to reduce their diet GI without drastically altering the nature of their diets merely by selecting specific brands or modifying food preparation methods.

For the interested reader, a GI database of over 400 foods is available at http://www.glycemicindex.com/. We encourage our clients to monitor their daily GI intake and consult GI cookbooks, including those listed below, to help facilitate weight loss and weight management:

- *The New Glucose Revolution: Low GI Eating Made Easy* by Jennie Brand-Miller, Kaye Foster-Powell, and Phillipa Sandall (2005).
- *The Low GI Diet Cookbook: 100 Simple, Delicious Smart-Carb Recipes—The Proven Way to Lose Weight and Eat for Lifelong Health (Glucose Revolution)* by Jennie Brand-Miller, Kay Foster-Powell, & Joanna McMillan-Price. (2005).
- *The New Glucose Revolution Shopper's Guide to GI Values 2008: The Authoritative Source of Glycemic Index Value for More than 1000 Foods* by Jennie Brand-Miller, Kaye Foster-Powell, and Fiona Atkinson (2007).

Another issue with glycemic index that must be considered is that some foods may have a higher GI, yet have good nutritional value that we won't want to pass up on. Carrots for instance do not have a low GI but they have good nutritional value. Glycemic index is based on all food weighing the same dry weight. Therefore, if you have a food that is somewhat higher in GI but has good nutritional value, such as a carrot, there is no need to be concerned about the GI value.

Food: When, Where, and How

To Graze or Not to Graze

There is some research that says that grazing, or eating smaller amounts over the course of a day, is better and healthier than eating three square meals a day. In a study published in the *International Journal of Obesity and Related Metabolic Disorders* (Speechly, Rogers, & Buffenstein,1999) one group of overweight men was given five small meals, then was free to choose a sixth meal. A second group ate a single meal containing the same number of calories as the total of the other group's first five meals, then later had a free-choice second meal. The six-meal men ate 27% less food at their last meal than the two-meal men did at their second. We typically encourage our clients to consume smaller meals more frequently, though we do so with caution as the empirical data supporting this particular dietary habit is equivocal. Further, knowing we are working with individuals who have "control" issues when eating, we run the risk of encouraging binge-type eating and this is certainly something we want to avoid. Therefore, we recommend that if you plan to encourage your clients to consume smaller, though more frequent meals, ensure that they are doing so with the right kinds of foods that tend to be low in GI and higher in nutritional value.

Speed Kills

Americans epitomize fast-food feasting. Drive through any suburb and throw a rock and you will likely hit one of several fast-food establishments. And if a fast-food burger, burrito, fish fillet, or roast beef sandwich isn't your thing, most gas stations have grab-and-go food available in their mini-marts. Oversized burgers, extra-large servings of fries, and buckets of soda, all at low prices, are enticing for the person on the run. Busy and cash-strapped families increasingly rely on take-out food for family dinners, and regular consumption of oversized portions of fatty foods has led to widespread obesity throughout the country. To put it bluntly, the prevalence of obesity, like America's waistband, seems to have no limits to its expansiveness.

In contrast, our neighbors across the Atlantic Ocean consume hearty portions of tasty food, now commonly referred to as the Mediterranean Diet, that hasn't put their health on the line. Defining a Mediterranean-style diet can be challenging, given the broad geographical region, including at least 16 countries, that borders the Mediterranean Sea. As would be expected, there are cultural, ethnic, religious, economic, and agricultural production differences that result in different dietary practices in these areas that preclude a single definition of a Mediterranean-style diet. Nonetheless, there is a dietary pattern that is characteristic of Mediterranean-style diets. This pattern emphasizes a diet that is high in fruits, vegetables, bread, cereals, potatoes, beans, nuts, and seeds. It also includes olive oil as an important fat source while restricting saturated and trans fats. Dairy products, fish, and poultry are consumed in low to moderate amounts, whereas there is little consumption of red meat, and eggs are consumed zero to four times weekly. In addition, wine (usually red) is consumed in low to moderate amounts.

There is provocative evidence from the Lyon Heart Study (de Lorgeril et al., 1999) suggesting that a Mediterranean-style diet is superior to the Western-style diet (i.e., lower caloric/fat/carbohydrate intake) typically recommended by American physicians and dieticians for weight loss, lowering cardiovascular risk, and minimizing obesity.

It has been postulated that Western Europeans enjoy healthier and less obese bodies, not only because of what, but how they eat. The French in particular have been recognized as taking time to enjoy their meals because they perceive meals as important relaxing social events. It has consequently been espoused by many dietary experts that slower eating leads to faster satiety and thus positively impacts weight management and/or weight loss. Though this notion seems very plausible, there is little and at times inconsistent empirical data to support it (Andrade, Greene, & Melanson, 2008). It does seem, however, that recent research suggests that the French, more so than Americans, rely on internal cues versus external cues for meal cessation, offering a partial explanation of why BMI might vary across people and cultures (Wansink, Payne, & Chandon, 2007).

In a study evaluating the effects of increasing portion size of foods on increased intake energy, Rolls, Roe, and Meeng discovered a direct relationship between portion size and overall consumption of food and possibly increased body weight (Rolls, Roe, & Meengs, 2006). By the same token, these same authors noted that reductions in portion size and energy density of food independently deceased free feeding behavior. These studies combined suggest that managing the portion size of food could have a direct impact on weight gain or weight loss.

Interestingly, the same is true of increased beverage consumption during meals. Flood and his colleagues (2006) examined the impact of increasing beverage portion size on beverage and food intake and noted that larger beverage portions results in increased beverage and food intake when a caloric beverage was served. In contrast, increased intake of low-calorie (or better yet, noncaloric) beverages appears to be an effective strategy for decreasing overall energy intake, thereby reducing overall consumption of food, because these drinks did not increase total energy consumed at a meal.

Another crucial component to food consumption has been referred to as *mindless eating*. Essentially, mindless eating amounts to relying on visual or other external environmental cues instead of internal feelings of satiety to determine when one is finished eating. Cornell University's Brian Wansink's award-winning academic research on food psychology and behavior change has been published in the some of the world's top marketing, medical, and nutrition journals. His ingenious research has contributed to the introduction of smaller "100 calorie" packages (to prevent overeating), the use of taller glasses in some bars (to prevent the overpouring of alcohol), and the use of elaborate names and mouth-watering descriptions on some chain restaurant menus (to improve enjoyment of the food).

Wansink has also been credited with determining that substituting a 10-inch dinner plate for a 12-inch plate results in 22% less food consumption (Wansink, 2004), that low-fat labels lead people to eat 16 to 23% more total calories (Wansink & Chandon, 2006), and that a person will eat an average of 92% of what they serve themselves (Wansink & Cheney, 2005).

Perhaps best known for his study using slowly and imperceptibly refilling soup bowls, Wansink, Painter, and North (2005) found that people tend to eat with their eyes and not their stomachs. Interestingly, Wansink noted that subjects in the "bottomless" bowl group consumed 73% more soup than their control group counterparts, yet did not believe they had consumed more, nor did they perceive themselves as more satiated than those eating from normal bowls. These findings are consistent with the notion that the amount of food on a plate or bowl increases intake because it influences consumption norms and expectations and it lessens one's reliance on self-monitoring.

Time Matters Not: Snack Smart!

Popular opinion, as unscientifically determined by a Google search of available information and opinions on the matter, suggests that late-night snacking leads to weight gain. The following Web sites cautioned against late-night eating, maintaining that the "extra" calories consumed before bedtime will add extra pounds that are likely unwanted: The Mayo Clinic at www.mayoclinic.com; The Colleagean, a student-maintained Web site at Penn State University at www.collegean.psu.com; and The American College of Sports Medicine at www.acsm.com.

It should be noted, however, that this same Google search revealed a number of studies debunking this now understood myth concerning nighttime eating. More specifically, research involving rhesus monkeys indicates that when food is consumed has far less impact on weight gain than *what and how much* one eats (Sullivan, Daniels, Koegler, & Cameron, 2005). These authors discerned that increased caloric intake for a group of female rhesus monkeys did not lead to weight gain over the course of one year when compared to another group of monkeys who were fed an equivalent amount of food during the day. Unexpectedly, this study also found that caloric intake did not specifically correlate with weight gain.

In a follow-up study, some of these same authors concluded that physical activity is a particularly important factor contributing to weight gain in adulthood and, when considered in isolation, may be more important for weight gain/loss than caloric intake alone (Sullivan, Koegler, & Cameron, 2006).

Although it is apparent that nighttime eating does not have as direct an impact upon weight gain as was once thought, there is evidence that this behavior impedes desired weight loss (Gluck, Geliebter, & Satov, 2001). Consequently, we do encourage our clients to consume most of their caloric daily intake several hours before bedtime. If they chose to eat later in the evening, we suggest they make wise choices by eating healthier foods that tend to have a lower glycemic index and higher nutritional value.

With the aforementioned data in mind, we offer the following suggestions to our clients for facilitating weight loss/management:

1. Keep a journal of all foods consumed for 2 to 3 weeks that indentifies what was eaten, how much was eaten, and when and where the food was consumed. This allows your clients and you to have a better understanding of their dietary habits. We also have our clients identify when they ate due to stress, boredom, or any other emotional situation that warrants attention.
2. Evaluate to the best extent possible, the glycemic index of most foods consumed.
3. Reduce total caloric consumption by 500 to 1,000 calories/day. Doing so will result in 1 to 2 pounds of weight loss in 1 week.
4. Reducing portions of food by using smaller plates or bowls.
5. Preloading some meals with noncaloric drinks like water or dietary soft drinks in limited quantity. Drinking water with a meal will also reduce energy intake and thereby influence overall food consumption.
6. Preload meals with fruit (e.g., apples in particular), as it has been shown to reduce energy intake, causing faster satiety and reduced consumption (Flood-Obbagy & Rolls, 2008).
7. Avoid alcoholic beverages before or during meals. As noted above, drinking caloric beverages before or during meals increases the likelihood that more food will be consumed.
8. Eat slower and more conscientiously.

FEAR OF FAT

Anticipated weight gain associated with smoking cessation tends to be a deterrent for quitting smoking. Most people who quit smoking gain, on average, between 5.5 and 15 pounds in the long term (Kawachi, Troisi, Rotnitzky, Coakley, & Colditz, 1996; Parsons, Shraim, Inglis, Aveyard, & Hajek, 2009). However, it is clear that the substantial health benefits of smoking cessation exceed the health complications associated with secondary weight gain. Furthermore, there is evidence to suggest that weight gain associated with smoking cessation occurs in selective individuals and can be minimized. Italian researchers Cairella et al., (2007) found that 52% of former smokers reported weight gain and, among these, 25.4% reported a weight gain of more than 10 pounds. They also found a direct association between female gender, age (45 to 65), and number of cigarettes smoked per day (more than 20/day) and weight gain after smoking cessation.

It is popularly believed that smoking decreases body weight by suppressing appetite. However, cross-sectional studies show that, despite their lower body weights, smokers do not eat less than nonsmokers or ex-smokers and, in fact, tend to eat slightly more (Perkins, 1992). Similarly, laboratory studies show no acute effects of smoking or nicotine intake via other means on caloric intake in smokers, although intake of nonsmokers may be reduced after nicotine exposure in women who have elevated BMI (Saules, Pomerleau, Snedecor, Brouwer, & Rosenberg, 2004).

In contrast, longitudinal studies show that eating consistently increases in the first weeks after stopping smoking, but may recede to pre-cessation levels with longer-term abstinence, whereas resumption of smoking after cessation is accompanied by a reduction in eating. (Mizoue, Ueda, Tokui, Hino, & Yoshimura, 1998). Thus, there appear to be no acute or chronic effects of smoking on eating in smokers maintaining regular smoking, but changes in eating are observed concomitant with changes in smoking status (i.e., cessation or relapse), though weight gain is not necessarily inevitable (Perkins, 1993).

Reducing caloric intake, increasing physical activity, and use of nicotine gum (Filozof, Fernandez Pinilla, & Fernandez-Cruz, 2004) have been shown to minimize unwanted weight gain following smoking cessation (Kawachi et al., 1996; Williamson et al., 1991).

Consistent with the empirical data reviewed above, many clients express concerns about weight gain secondary to quitting smoking and initially resist suggestions that they consider a smoking cessation program. It has been our experience, however, that providing our clients with accurate information (including the published articles themselves, especially for individuals whose Enneagram results suggest personalities within the Thinking Triad) regarding possible weight gain secondary to smoking cessation enhances their motivation to become permanent nonsmokers. Further, encouraging and facilitating dietary changes and increased physical activity during a smoking cessation program allows our clients to minimize weight gain, and in some cases, to lose weight.

It should be noted that one challenge we confront as providers helping clients become permanent nonsmokers is the general lifestyle of smokers. Smokers tend to be less physically active, engage in more sedentary activities like watching television or surfing the Internet, and consume less than five servings of fruits and vegetables per day compared with nonsmokers (Strine et al., 2005).

In an effort to facilitate a permanently nonsmoking, fit-and-trim lifestyle, we focus on six strategies to break the connection between smoking and weight gain because it is a concern for many of our clients. For some clients, we may spend more or less time on any one or more of the six strategies, depending upon the circumstances in their life. For instance, if our client is physically fit and exercises regularly, despite being a smoker, we would spend far less time discussing exercise and perhaps focus more time and energy on stress management strategies. As emphasized throughout this book, it is important to individualize treatment and not approach each client with the same, "cookie-cutter" program.

Six Considerations for Breaking the Smoking–Weight Gain Dilemma

1. Weigh the options.
2. Manage the stress.
3. Reward within reason.
4. Mind your metabolism.
5. Fix the oral fixation.
6. Heal thyself with health.

Weigh the Options

Many smokers who consider a nonsmoking lifestyle have understandable concerns about gaining weight. Knowing this, we take time to address the benefits of becoming permanent nonsmokers and contrast that with the possibility of gaining unwanted weight. As discussed previously, some clients will readily absorb this information, weigh the options and, with our assistance, initiate a plan that minimizes weight gain. Presenting them with the black-and-white evidence of the benefits of not smoking, the risks of smoking, and accurate scientific data regarding possible weight gain associated with quitting smoking, we find that most people become motivated to do that which is in their best health interests.

Manage the Stress

No one is immune to stress. It has been credited with generating physical illness like migraine headaches, ulcers, and hypertension and either directly or indirectly contributing to many causes of preventable death, including cancer, strokes, diabetes, and heart attacks. Many smokers continue to smoke, believing it helps manage stress while giving them a sense of calm that they otherwise lack in life. For these individuals, we offer alternative ways to manage stress, including a reasonable exercise regimen, and relaxation strategies like progressive muscle relaxation, yoga, or meditation. Instead of putting cigarettes in their mouths, we encourage them to find other, healthier behaviors that can manage stress.

Reward Within Reason

There is ample evidence proving beyond any reasonable doubt that human beings are motivated by rewards. Parents and preschools employ token economies to condition positive behavior. Companies utilize hourly pay rates, incentives based on productivity, and salaries, all of which are grounded in principles of positive reinforcement schedules. At times, we implement our own personal reward system that acknowledges accomplishment. We celebrate with others and reward them for living another year by sharing cake and candles. A job promotion, acquisition of a new job, major life transition, or Hallmark Holiday will frequently include a celebratory meal or special food treat. When smokers become permanent nonsmokers, we encourage them to reward or reinforce themselves in ways that do not involve food. During the treatment process, and usually earlier than later, we have our clients identify things that motivate them or activities that they enjoy. We have them calculate the amount of money they will save in one, two, or three months by not smoking and suggest they identify something else they can spend that money on. Some clients simply choose to save their money before determining something they want to purchase. As long as they have a history suggesting success using delayed gratification, we tell them to go for it.

Mind Your Metabolism

Smoking does indeed increase one's metabolism. Unfortunately, it also raises blood pressure, heart rate, and carbon monoxide (a colorless, odorless, tasteless deadly gas) levels. Of course there are healthier ways to increase metabolism, like aerobic and anaerobic exercise, or resistance training with free weights (Dolezal & Potteiger, 1998). Though some studies (e.g., Wilmore et al., 1998) failed to find a significant correlation between resting metabolic rate (RMR) and resistance training, Speakman and Selman (2003) in their extensive review of relevant published studies noted that long-term effects of training increase RMR. These authors also noted that studies which failed to find a significant relationship between resistance training and RMR were potentially confounded by an experimental design that failed to account for longer-term effects of training on RMR. This effect of resistance training on RMR seems to be more prominent for men than for women, though additional benefits of weight training are noted regardless of gender (Lemmer et al., 2001).

In general, most studies employing resistance training utilized techniques espoused by body-building guru Joe Weider (e.g., pyramid principle, split training system, progressive overload principle). It has been our experience that most of our clients have not been exposed to resistance training and have little knowledge of the correct and incorrect ways to lift weights. Most fitness centers have trainers available to offer assistance to the novice weight trainer. For individuals who plan to purchase their own equipment, whether that involves a few free weights or complicated weight training machines, we encourage them to educate themselves about proper weight-lifting techniques, so as to minimize injury and maximize gains. Instructional material is readily available in print media (e.g., *Muscle and Fitness, Men's Fitness, Men's Health, Muscle and Fitness Hers, Shape*) or online references (www.weight-training.realsolutionsmag.com or www.muscleandfitness.com).

Fix the Oral Fixation

Though many theories have come under attack over the years, perhaps one that has stood the test of time is the notion of oral fixations. According to Freud, "The first organ to emerge as an erotogenic zone and to make libidinal demands on the mind is, from the time of birth onwards, the mouth. To begin with, all psychical activity is concentrated on providing satisfaction for the needs of that zone. Primarily, of course, this satisfaction serves the purpose of self-preservation by means of nourishment; but physiology should not be confused with psychology.

The baby's obstinate persistence in sucking gives evidence at an early stage of a need for satisfaction which, though it originates from and is instigated by the taking of nourishment, nevertheless strives to obtain pleasure independently of nourishment and for that reason may and should be termed sexual" (1949, p. 24).

The primary conflict at this stage of development is the weaning process such that the child must become less dependent upon caretakers. If fixation occurs at this stage, Freud maintained that the individual would have issues with dependency or aggression. Hence, an oral fixation can result, manifesting behaviorally as uncontrolled drinking, eating, smoking, or nail biting.

Heal Thyself With Health

By this we mean assuming the identity of a health-oriented person. For many people who smoke and/or are overweight, the notion of perceiving themselves as healthy is foreign and likely has been for quite some time. This new perspective consequently involves a shift in lifestyle that requires adjustments in diet, exercise, and general well-being, including sleep, alcohol consumption, and minimization of sedentary activities. When people perceive themselves as healthy, as living a lifestyle that enhances their quality of life, they are less likely to engage in behaviors that are physically self-destructive. Throughout this text, we emphasize the importance of becoming a permanent nonsmoker and/or permanently fit and trim. It isn't about going *on* a diet to later come *off* a diet, or initiating an exercise program to reach an end goal for the exercise program to conclude. Rather, our focus is on life-changing behaviors that involve permanence.

CONCLUSION

In this chapter, we reviewed the importance of providing our clients with accurate information regarding the adverse effects of obesity and smoking and the immediate and long-term health implications of becoming a permanent nonsmoker and permanently fit and trim. We discussed the importance of basal metabolic rate and offered an Internet link that provides a BMI calculator. Although the glycemic index has its limitations for determining the quality of food consumed, it does offer assistance and guidelines that permit guidance with implementing a healthier diet to promote weight loss.

It is important to monitor not only what kind of food is consumed, but how it is consumed as well. For example, in this chapter we reviewed recent empirical studies that underscore the importance of smaller portion size, how perception may override internal sensation of satiety, and how speed of consumption can influence the amount of food eaten.

Finally we address the challenges that we may confront when working with smokers who are concerned about gaining unwanted weight. We offered five strategies for addressing these obstacles and how we can help smokers become permanent nonsmokers who gain little if any weight during the initial phases of their smoking cessation program.

Things to Do

1. Review with a client information regarding the benefits of not smoking and the changes that can occur within the body soon after the last cigarette is smoked (see Table 5.1).
2. Encourage one of your clients desiring a more fit and trim body to implement any of the eight recommendations reviewed above, including calculating the glycemic index of food consumed.
3. Review the reference material provided above concerning resistance training, particularly if you are not familiar with concepts such as the pyramid principle, split training, and the progressive muscle overload principle.

6 Begin With the End in Mind: Setting Well-Formed Goals

In the absence of clearly-defined goals, we become strangely loyal to performing daily trivia until ultimately we become enslaved by it.

—*Robert Heinlein*

THREE RULES FOR CREATING WELL-FORMED GOALS

First, we believe that goals should be framed in positive terms. Surely you have encountered clients who, when asked to state their personal goals for therapy, have done so in terms of what they *do not* want rather than what they *do* want. Perhaps they say, "I don't want to lose my temper" or "I don't want to be fat" or "I don't want to be anxious or nervous anymore." We can reframe these goals in more positive terms by helping our clients define what they do want. So for instance, we may ask, "If you don't want to be fat, what do you want to be?" or "If you were not wanting to be overweight, what would you be doing to lose weight?" or "If you did not lose your temper, what would you be doing instead?"

Goals should also be concrete and measurable and not vague or amorphous so that there is no way of knowing whether the goal is being reached or not. Without measureable goals, we have no way of knowing whether we are making progress and whether the interventions we have utilized are of benefit.

Finally, accomplishing the goal should be within the client's control. Goals that are not achievable or within an individual's control are likely to be met with failure and frustration.

Connecting Your Client's Ideal Self To Her Future Self

Before initiating any treatment plan, it is important to have an understanding of what the goal will look like. Because the unconscious mind knows how to structure and understand the difference between present, past, and future, we employ trance work to connect an individual's ideal self to their future self. Thus we begin in the present by having people project into their future and begin to see, feel, and experience the self they want to be.

To help our clients connect to their ideal selves, we help them amplify and empower the experience during trance work. We want a trance to have high impact, as our experience has shown that doing so enhances the potential for making the connection between the client's ideal self and future self. With the assistance of hypnosis, we bring our clients' ideal selves to life by using vivid and compelling images that motivate them to embrace their ideal selves and maintain a level of motivation to make the necessary changes in their lives to become permanent nonsmokers or become permanently fit and trim.

If we are to help our clients appreciate the permanence of their decision to change unwanted habits, we also have to introduce an element of inevitability. Before consulting with you, your clients have likely tried and failed many programs, diets, and/or exercise regimens or purchased exercise equipment that now serves as a place to dry wet clothes. Knowing there have been attempts and likely failures (though some successes, which have not been permanent), it is important to encode a sense of inevitability in our treatment.

There are a number of procedures and strategies that we employ with our clients to create this inevitability. Whereas some people are very good at using imagery, others are not. Therefore, we want to use more than just hypnotic imagery to help our clients impart a sense of inevitability to their desire to change their unwanted habit permanently.

First, we ask our clients to point to a place in front of them where they can imagine seeing their new goal-image, "the permanently slim and fit Jim or Sally" or "Jim/Sally the permanent nonsmoker." Most people will readily imagine this person and point to a place in space where they can imagine the new person being. It may be to their left, their right, or directly in front of them. For individuals encountering difficulty with this exercise, in particular people who may say they aren't able to imagine or perceive anything, we ask them to imagine someone they like and someone they don't like. We then ask them to identify each person by name and let us know when they have a solid image of both people in mind. Once they confirm this for us, we then ask "Who is on the left?" They will then identify one of the people, which then allows us to help them understand how they can take an image from inside their mind and project it somewhere out in space.

Once the person appreciates how he is able to do this, we then ask him to see the permanently slim "you" or the permanent nonsmoking "you" and have him point to that person. We never ask if the client can see his future self, we simply presuppose that he can and ask the client to identify where he sees himself.

For those rare individuals who continue to have difficulty with this imagery, we take a step back and have them begin to imagine something with less emotional attachment. Perhaps their car, or home, or backyard, or a football game they watched. We then encourage them to close their eyes and describe everything to us. If necessary, we may cue them by asking "Does the car have a scratch on it anywhere?" or "Does the grass in your yard need to be cut?" or "Have you ever noticed how your yard has different shades of green because of the different kinds of grass that are in it?"

After we have reasonable confidence that they can image the individual they want to be, we have them project it into their future—amplified, empowered, and coded with inevitability by the very words we use and the imagery we suggest.

Creating A Path Between Your Client and the Client's Future Self

After an image has been vividly created, we introduce the notion of a path between the person the client is at this moment and the person she wants to be. We help the client understand that this is a path that she will move along and in so doing come closer to connecting with her desired self. Doing so allows our client to have a greater sense of security that there is a process that we are following and that she is part of this process and moving toward the goal.

We then discuss the elements of the plan that we intend to implement with them along this path. At this time we may mention hypnosis or self-hypnosis, or if you prefer relaxation and imagery. If the primary concern involves food, we mention plans to address and recommend healthy dietary choices and effective exercise regimens that do not have to create pain and discomfort for maximum benefit.

Knowing that many habits involve automatic, seemingly unconscious behaviors, we help our clients interrupt the connections that have developed over time and reinforced the unwanted behavior. For instance, for the smoker, we encourage them to smoke with their opposite hand, or keep cigarettes in an inconvenient place that forces them to seek them out elsewhere rather than a shirt pocket or purse. For one client, David encouraged him to put his cigarettes at the top of his kitchen cabinet, where he had to stand on a step-stool every time he wanted to smoke a cigarette. For automobile smokers, we recommend they keep their cigarettes in the trunk of their car. Though the backseat or glove box may be inconvenient enough, they pose hazards for the driver who is determined to get a cigarette even if it means temporarily taking his hands off the wheel. By keeping the cigarettes in the trunk of the car, the client must pull over and get out of the car to get to a cigarette.

Many smokers associate smoking with other behaviors, such as drinking a cup of coffee, or sitting at a bar sipping at a cocktail. For the coffee-smoker, we suggest tea instead, and in a different location. For the smoker who has a cigarette after eating, we suggest a walk or other activity that precludes smoking. Sometimes, simply changing the brand of preferred cigarettes helps a smoker break the cycle that has been established over the years.

For individuals encountering difficulties changing their dietary behaviors, we encourage them to shop at a different grocery store, or allow someone else in the home (if they exist) who may be a more conscientiously healthy shopper make the trip to the store instead. Or if, on the contrary, someone else in the house manages the grocery shopping and brings home unhealthy foods, we empower our client to take over this chore and gain greater control over the food products that enter her home. Like the smoker who is encouraged to smoke with the opposite hand, we suggest the same for the client who desires a more fit and healthy body. Eating with the opposite hand also has a way of slowing down food consumption, which in turn may permit satiety before overeating has occurred. Additionally, knowing that many of our clients live on a fast-food diet, we encourage them to plan and shop ahead before they are restricted to fast-food choices because their time to eat is limited. This becomes particularly challenging for clients who either live, work, or go to school in neighborhoods where there is a disproportionate number of fast-food restaurants. Davis and Carpenter (2008) found that students with fast-food restaurants within one-half mile of their schools consumed fewer servings of fruits and vegetables, consumed more servings of soda, and were more likely to be overweight or obese than were youths whose schools were not near fast-food restaurants.

For clients who work in environments where unhealthy food is readily available, we encourage them to move the food as far away from their workstation as possible. Though this seems to be a trivial matter, Wansink, Painter, and Lee (2006) observed that people ate an average of 2.2 more pieces of candy each day when the candy was visible, and 1.8 more pieces when they were proximately placed on their desk rather than 2 meters away.

We will also include in this plan new strategies using Energy Psychology for unblocking longstanding obstacles, reducing and controlling unwanted urges, and minimizing stress and anxiety that promotes unwanted behaviors.

Like any plan that involves personal change, a sense of commitment is necessary for the change to take place. In an effort to promote and enable commitment, we ask our clients if they believe they are dependable and able to keep commitments. Like most people who perceive themselves to be average or better-than-average drivers, most people also believe themselves to be dependable and very good at keeping commitments. (Truth be told, most people probably identify themselves as above average or excellent drivers, which of course is statistically impossible. But there is no need to point this out to a client who is trying to change!)

After asking our client about her capacity to make a commitment, we invite her to close her eyes, consider the last commitment she made to someone else and how empowering that felt, and then consider making a commitment to *himself* with as much integrity and importance as she would to someone else. We then validate the experience for the client, reinforcing her ability to not only make a commitment, but keep it, especially with himself or herself, *no matter what.*

Putting It to Music

Because we want our clients' experience to be empowered in all sensory systems, we have them consider their journey as if it were a movie, a movie of them moving down a path of becoming the person they want to be. Because movies are scored and orchestrated, we have them select a song that will be their theme song. Most people have no difficulty identifying with a theme song and most of those songs are motivating, and have a driving beat that fosters an image of success (e.g., the film *Rocky*). At times, however, we may have some clients who select soothing songs like *Pachelbel's Canon.* We encourage such clients to consider something that will be more likely to propel them into action than calm them to such a degree that they may fall asleep! After they have identified their theme song, we tell them to play it while imagining themselves moving down the path to success, becoming the permanent nonsmoker or permanently fit person they desire to be. Of course they can have several theme songs if they wish. Some of our clients maintain a soundtrack, as it were, that permits a variety of songs to inspire and motivate them to stay true to their commitment.

The Gift

The technique we call "The Gift," like any gift one receives in life, serves to reinforce and motivate. With habit control, the gift is a way of summarizing their experience, of developing a healthy self-image, of solidifying their goal-image and showing them what a great gift this is that they can give to themselves. We present the gift during a semihypnotic trance. If you prefer, it can be with the same eye closure as you used for the "having commitment"—just having the person in this state and saying to them, "What a gift this new you, this new self-image, this new goal-image is for you."

After ensuring that our client is experiencing a comfortable trance, we encourage him to consider how his mind is able to grasp the concept of inevitability. For instance, we all "know" that tomorrow morning the sun will rise and later in the day will set. Although we all have hopes and aspirations, some of them may not be inevitable. For example, you may play the Lotto, *knowing* you are not likely to win and yet *hoping* you will. We have our clients play these images out in their minds and identify a place out in space where they can point to the inevitable sunrise, and another place for the not-likely-to-happen Lotto win. Then we have them notice how big and bright the image of the sunrise is while that of the lottery is dimmer, not as clear, not as close. Using "hypnotic" images like *bigger, closer, stronger,* we are setting the stage for our client's mind to encode the inevitable. After ensuring that our client grasps this concept, having a three-dimensional, detailed, and colorful image of a sunrise in mind, we have the client include a picture of himself as the permanently slim and fit person he wants to be. We have the client include this three-dimensional image of his future self in conjunction with that of the inevitable sunset. Having this image in mind, we then leave an open-ended suggestion of inevitability by saying, "Once you have this image clearly in mind, as you look at this John, I want you to say in your most persuasive positive voice, 'This shall be.' " By having the client determine *when* he will say these words (rather than us telling him when to say them), we are essentially using presupposition. We have presupposed that the client will be able to see this image of his future self and, once he utters the words, "This shall be," the client validates the experience.

It is important to emphasize certain words for our clients during trance experiences. That emphasis should have a sense of confidence in the inevitability of these words. We tell them, "Look at *this* Judy, the *permanently slim and fit* Judy. *This* Judy is the gift of the quality and quantity of life that you desire. *She* is the gift of improved health and freedom from disease, a gift of more energy and vitality, wearing the clothes you want to wear, hearing the compliments from others that validate the slim and fit Judy. This is who you *really are* inside and *will soon be* fully experiencing in your life, now and always."

CONCLUSION

In this chapter, we reviewed the importance of beginning with the end in mind. By working with our clients to identify desired goals in positive terms, we help them establish concrete and achievable goals. Understanding that habits are driven by both conscious and unconscious behavior, we offered a number of environmental and behavioral recommendations that involve more conscious deliberation and choices. By including hypnotic strategies or guided imagery, we help our clients access and mobilize resources that would otherwise be neglected and unused. Using the image of a path that includes a sense of inevitability, we encourage them to put their "movie" to music, as music can be personally inspiring and motivating. Finally, we introduced the concept of commitment by introducing "The Gift" via hypnotic imagery. It has been our experience that including The Gift with vivid images of inevitability and inviting verbalization, including "this shall be," enhances a client's commitment to her goal or goals.

Things to Do

1. Work with a client and help him/her identify a treatment goal or revisit the goal you identified at the end of chapter 1. Go through the process or have your client go through the process of imagining the goal and describing the goal in detail.
2. Select a theme song and listen to it while imagining the goal that you or your client desires.
3. With a client or by yourself, consider the gift that is received, experiencing it in its inevitability, without doubt, no matter what.

7   Homework: It's Not Just for Children

For homework tonight, write in your journal section about how your dreams now will determine your future success.

—Jean Webb

Thus far, we have laid out a process for conducting a habit assessment, gathering useful information from the Enneagram that can guide treatment, and building a sequence of interventions seeking reasons for change that facilitate permanent habit control. Because purpose drives motivation, our treatment frequently includes a review of progress and goals and revisits reasons for making changes through relevant medical information, as discussed in chapter 5. Additionally, we emphasized the importance of moving from an intellectual understanding of the benefits of habit control to having personal experiences of these benefits, so that a client's new goal-image becomes compelling, inviting, and magnetic. Through this entire process, it is well-formulated homework assignments that allow our clients to move down the path that begins in the present and leads them in the direction of becoming a permanent nonsmoker and/or permanently fit and trim. We generally encourage some homework assignment of one kind or another after each session, as it has been our experience that these assignments offer a catalyst for continued change and progress.

FIVE ACTIVITIES AND ASSIGNMENTS TO PROMOTE HABIT CONTROL

1. Become Very Good Friends With Your Future Self

After helping our client gain a new self-image that is more compelling, magnetic, and inviting, we then introduce what we refer to as "The Gift," and eventually hypnosis, to reinforce the client's goal of permanent habit control. Typically, we invite our client to close his eyes and, after discussing the gift, we gently encourage the client to become very good friends with *this Stephen*, "because *this Stephen* is really who you are and who you will now be fully manifesting in your life." We then ask our client to "Let *this Stephen* guide, direct, and influence your behaviors and choices. What would *this Stephen* do? How would *this new Stephen*, the permanent nonsmoker, find new ways of marking out time? How will *Stephen-the-permanent-nonsmoker* enjoy all the increasing energy and vitality?"

If the client is religious, we might also say, "You know, there are some Christians who wear bracelets that read WWJD, What Would Jesus Do? and you might want to think about WWSD, What Would this Stephen Do?" Of course, we are very mindful about who we say something like this to, as some Christians may be offended by the notion that their name might replace that of Jesus in the WWJD phrase or even (if non-Christian) be offended by the mere mention of Jesus.

Realize, when working with our clients, we are not telling them what to do or what not to do. We are not directly telling them, "You have to stop smoking," or "You have to lose weight this week." Rather, we are preparing them and initiating a process without generating conflict, stress, or a sense of perfectionism. We are encouraging them to become really good friends with *this Stephen,* asking them to let this *future Stephen* guide, direct, and influence their behaviors and choices. Knowing that most of our clients have self-esteem issues that can interfere with treatment progress when frustration sets in because they are not losing the weight they want to lose or not cutting back on their cigarette smoking, we help the client get in touch with his or her future self, who is already successful. It is *that Stephen* who will be making the good decisions that allow him to continue down the path of being *Stephen-the-permanent-nonsmoker.* Instead of us *pushing* the client down a path of becoming a permanent nonsmoker, we want his future self to *pull* him toward the person he wants to be.

2. The Benefits and Traps of Willpower

At times, clients struggling to make changes may tell us that their primary problem is that they lack willpower. Though it may be tempting to help them find that willpower to help them engage in treatment, we generally tell our clients that a lack of willpower is not necessarily a bad thing. When someone relies on willpower alone to propel change, it tells us that he or she is not aligned with her future self. Ultimately, clients who are "waiting on willpower" to promote the change they seek are struggling with a desire to continue to smoke or overeat or not engage in physical activities that promote weight loss. We know that willpower alone is not adequate for facilitating and maintaining change. And if a client has willpower, but hasn't internalized and integrated a sense of comfortable change that leads her down the path of being a permanent nonsmoker, her initial desire to manage unwanted behaviors is likely to fade over time.

3. Check the Superego at the Door

It is very important from time to time to remind your clients to keep their superegos under control, as the superego can and will interfere with treatment progress. The role of the superego is to aim for perfection and strive to act in a socially appropriate manner. It operates our sense of right and wrong, is fueled by guilt, and develops out of early parental interjections and injunctions, rules, and regulations which have been added to by society, religion, schools, and so on. By its very nature, the superego is rigid because it is of the past and does not strive to guide behavior on the basis of compassion, awareness, or being present.

As odd as it may seem, harsh superegos can perpetually reinforce and maintain unwanted habits. At first glance you might think the superego would help harness uncontrolled, unhealthy behaviors like smoking and overeating; however, it is the harshness of the superego to which the habit response is really unconsciously directed. Given all the pressures and stress of daily living and expectations to live and behave in certain ways in an effort to avoid the unwanted pressure from a critical and punitive society, people may overeat or smoke cigarettes to escape.

Even though the superego may aid an individual with controlling unwanted behaviors and unhealthy habits, we must use caution as therapists that we not reinforce the critical and self-abasing perspective of a harsh superego that promotes unhealthy behavior that offers temporary relief. Therefore well-planned homework assignments that promote greater levels of awareness and mindfulness to being-in-the-present can minimize the critical response from the superego, which operates in the past.

4. Preparing: Doing and Avoiding

It is at this point in the treatment process that we ask the client what he can begin doing that will further his progress. This involves putting the client into action by introducing and encouraging new behaviors while avoiding old behavioral patterns that either promote the unwanted behavior or have failed to control it. For instance, for the client who plays poker in a smoke-filled room every Thursday night, you may encourage this person to avoid this group for a few weeks. If you have a client who is planning to initiate an exercise program, now may be a good time for him to go to the gym and sign up for a membership.

Below is a list of recommendations we offer to our clients to prepare them for the changes ahead:

- Removing all ashtrays from the house
- Cleaning out the car
- Eliminating fattening, unhealthy food
- Shopping and preparing healthy foods/menu—Identify meals and food that you want to eat and set up a recipe book that will help you stay on track with your plans.
- Consider the people you will spend time with—do their habits challenge your plans?
- Consider the places you will go—what will you be doing (eating, smoking, drinking)?
- Change your environment (house, car, workspace, refrigerator, bedroom, bathroom) to support the "new" you—Display pictures, posters, or a list of all the reasons to be "Stephen, the permanent nonsmoker."

- Make a "public" announcement to solicit a support system and inform these people of your plans for making permanent changes in your life so that they won't inadvertently sabotage your plans. If you use Facebook or Twitter, make a public announce to gather support from friends, family, and other associates.
- Identify people you may need to avoid or limit contact with.
- Select a date to stop smoking or start an exercise program.
- Identify how much money you will save by not smoking and consider what you might spend that money on instead. Perhaps getting some brochures from places you'd like to visit, things you'd like to do, or finding a picture of something you'd like to purchase. (In 2009, the average cost for a pack of cigarettes was $4.50–$5.00, including taxes, depending on where a person lives. In 1 year, a pack-a-day smoker will save about $1,600. A 40-year-old who quits smoking and puts the savings into a 401(k) earning 9% a year would have nearly $250,000 by age 70. More precise figures including cumulative yearly savings can be determined by plugging in personal numbers based on your own smoking behavior at: http://www.bankrate.com/brm/cgi-bin/savings.asp.)

5. Record Keeping

When making a recommendation for your client to keep records, we must consider the purpose behind the assignment. Without a sense of purpose, record keeping becomes nothing more than busy work that in the end is likely to be abandoned. Though some clients may welcome and even initiate a detailed system using spreadsheets and data analysis for record keeping (see Enneagram Type 5 in chapter 3), others may not be inclined to put pen to paper even once to document behavioral patterns, as it seems a burden to their spontaneity. A one-size-fits-all approach is impractical; it is important to be mindful of your client and her desire, ability, and capacity to keep personal records. For some of our clients, we won't have them keep any records at all, as it will be distracting or burdensome, and may possibly interfere with treatment.

Record keeping offers people the opportunity to make a more objective examination of themselves and their behaviors. At times, our clients may say they are not certain why they smoke when they smoke. They perceive their behavior as simply spontaneous, without much fore-thought or conscious intention. It's just a habit, they will tell us, lacking any awareness of the triggers, cues, or precipitants to smoking a ciga-rette. Similarly, it is not uncommon for our clients to tell us that, despite being overweight, they don't eat much food, and that the food they eat isn't particularly unhealthy. Keeping records will allow these clients the opportunity to examine their habits more closely and make more informed and conscious decisions in the future.

For most of our clients, we have them keep daily records for a brief period of time. We ask them to note what they eat, when they eat, how they eat, or when they smoke and how much they smoke for a couple of weeks. If the client is finding that record keeping helps him stay true to himself, we encourage the client to continue with it. If, on the other hand, ample data is gathered to permit and promote change, the client doesn't have to continue with keeping daily records.

Realize that most people may not be the best record keepers or, even if they do record some data, may not identify the most relevant pieces of data, or may inaccurately record information, particularly if it is documented after the fact. For clients who will keep records, we ask them to write things either before or soon after they do them rather than at the end of the day or the following day. There is ample empirical data that overweight individuals underreport dietary consumption, par-ticularly if it is recorded 24 hours (or more) after consumption (see Jackson, Byrne, Magarey, & Hills, 2008; Novotny et al., 2003).

We therefore suggest that people record *before* or *immediately after* they eat. Doing so also has a second benefit, namely, that often people will consider what they have just documented, appreciate their caloric intake, and possibly curb their behavior for the remainder of the day. With the advent of Palm Pilots, PDAs, and smart phones, people can readily and conveniently maintain an accurate food-consumption diary.

After the data is recorded, we want to analyze it in ways that make a difference for the client. Again, we do not want this experience to be wasteful or an expenditure of time and energy for naught. We have our clients record information in ways that will help us help them. We generally take an entire session to review the recorded data, to look for themes and patterns, and to make sense of what the client has been doing that has been problematic so that we can correct the patterns of behavior and initiate effective interventions.

Knowing that people may grow tired of tedious record keeping, especially if they are not making the necessary changes in behavior and appreciating any benefit, we keep close tabs on how helpful the assignment is for them. We want to ensure that a sense of excitement and benefit is elicited from their efforts. Eventually, we want our clients to be able to intuitively monitor and calibrate their progress or lack thereof. An excessive reliance on record keeping does not generally bode well for permanent, internalized, and integrated habit control.

RECORD KEEPING: THE NUTS AND BOLTS

When it comes to record keeping, we want to ensure that we gather all the essential information necessary without generating overkill. In our experience, the following pieces of data are relevant and helpful with offering individualized recommendations:

- **When** does the behavior occur?
- **Where** does the behavior occur?
- With **whom** does the behavior occur?
- What **happened** just before the behavior occurred?
- What was the person **thinking** before, during, and after the behavior occurred?
- What was the person **feeling** before, during, and after the behavior occurred (bored, angry, sad, empty, anxious, lonely, etc.)?
- **How much** of the behavior occurred (caloric consumption, kind of food, number of cigarettes smoked)?

Using Charts

When our clients are interested in using charts, we print out the following charts for them to use. People are less likely to take the time to design their own chart, so we have one ready for them to use if they are interested. Again, not every client will use a chart. We generally show our clients the chart and then ask them if they would be interested in using one. Table 7.1 offers an example of what a daily food diary

Table 7.1

Daily Food Diary

Time	Food	Quantity	Calories	Emotions/Context	Hungry?	Result
8 am	Eggs, muffin, OJ, bacon	Medium	300	Just woke up.	Yes	Satiated.
10 am	6 Oreo cookies	Medium	610	Bored, lonely.	Not really	Guilty.
2 pm	Chips, ham and cheese sandwich, milk, more cookies	Medium	600	Alone, time for lunch, ate too fast.	Yes!	Too full.
3:15 pm	Chocolate cake, 2 scoops vanilla ice cream	Large	345	Bored, tired.	A little	Mad at self.
6:30 pm	Spaghetti, salad, ranch dressing, baked potato, three pieces of bread with butter	Medium	510	Very hungry, ate with husband.	Yes	Full, tired within 30 minutes. Probably overate.
11 pm	Cake	Large piece	200	Hungry, watching TV.	Not really	Empty.

may look like; Table 7.2 provides an example of a smoker's record for cigarettes smoked.

It is our experience that at least for the first 2 weeks of record keeping, we are able to gather ample data to help our clients gain a greater level of insight concerning their patterns of behavior that sustain their unwanted habits. For most clients, this is adequate, though some personalities will want to continue to monitor their behavior and use this data to assess their progress and modify their treatment plan if necessary. Others may revisit this data at a later date so that they can examine the progress made to date.

CONCLUSION

In this chapter, we reviewed the importance of well-selected homework assignments that not only put our clients in motion with regard to initiating behavior change but also establish an expectation of permanent habit control. In so doing, we discussed five important activities and assignments: becoming good friends with a future self, considering the importance of willpower, checking the superego, preparing for change, and record keeping. Promoting a relationship with one's future self helps clients become aligned with a sense of permanence and sets the expectation of change. Having a sense of self-respect also reduces the risk for future self-destructive behavior, including overeating and smoking.

As record keeping can be very helpful for allowing clients the opportunity to engage in a more objective self-assessment, provided of course the record keeping is accurate, we offered a number of options for how clients can keep track of their unwanted behaviors. Benefits and potential pitfalls of record keeping were considered when encouraging clients to keep daily diaries of their unwanted behaviors. Finally, at the close of this chapter, we provided examples of daily diaries for food consumption and smoking.

Things to Do

1. Encourage a client to engage in activities that foster a better relationship with their future self.

Table 7.2

Daily Smoking Diary

Time	Quantity	Emotions/Context	Urge	Result
6:30 am	2	Just woke up, smoke with cup of coffee in kitchen.	Strong	Felt relaxed.
8:10 am	3	Argument with wife, left for work, driving in car.	Very strong	Irritable before, during, after.
10 am	1	Took break from work.	Moderate	Calm.
11:15 am	2	Took break from work, smoked with coworker.	Mild to moderate	None really.
2:30 pm	3	Delivered package for work, driving in car.	Moderate	Relaxed.
3:30 pm	1	Took break from work, smoked alone.	Mild	Relaxed.
5:15 pm	3	Drove home from work.	Moderate	Initially relaxed, then stressed coming home.
6:10 pm	2	Smoked outside, expecting wife home from work.	Moderate, stressed about wife and possible arguments.	Stressed.
7:30 pm	2	Smoked outside, after dinner.	Mild	Relaxed.
10 pm	2	Before going to bed.	Mild	Upset that I didn't cut back today.

2. Have your client identify three or four interventions from the list provided in this chapter in an effort to engage her in treatment and promote an expectation of change.
3. Introduce record keeping to your client and, if he is interested and would likely benefit from it, have him keep a daily diary for at least 1 week. Review the data with your client to promote interventions that will address the pattern of behaviors that continues to promote unwanted behaviors.

May the Force Be With You

Do, or do not. There is no "try."
—Jedi Master Yoda

8   A History of Hypnosis

Your vision will only become clear when you look into your heart.... Who looks outside, dreams. Who looks inside awakens.

—Carl Jung

Hypnosis. What was your reaction when you first heard the word? Did you considered the power, magic, and mystery of the concept of hypnosis? Picture a shiny gold watch swaying before your trance-ready eyes? Perhaps you likened it to mind control? Age regression? Brain-washing? Or maybe the secret ability to mystically tap the unconscious mind to unearth buried skeletons haunting neurotic personalities? A kind of subconscious dumpster diving, if you will!

We pose these questions, silly as they may sound, because we believe it is important for you to recall your initial reaction to the word "hypnosis," as your personal experience could serve as a valuable reference when introducing your clients to one of the most—if not *the* most—misunderstood psychotherapeutic treatment intervention at our disposal as mental health professionals.

The word "hypnosis" has an aura of intrigue associated with it. For some, hypnosis is a welcome opportunity to relieve the emotional discomfort, physical pain, sleepless nights, and anxiety that plagues them. Others may tune in to their subconscious mind to improve athletic performance or ignite some motivation to propel themselves to successful endeavors. Others may question the authenticity and benefit of what for them is the unexplored territory of "tranceland." You will also, no doubt (pun intended), encounter the Doubting Thomas types who could never believe it until they see it. For these folks, David likes to encourage them to reconsider their perspective on hypnosis by adopting a "Believe it, then you'll see it" mind-set. Finally, we have those who, predominantly because of fear of the unknown or simpe ignorance, will resist the opportunity to give themselves the chance to benefit from hypnosis. Though fortunately representing a small minority of clients we have seen, you are likely to encounter the occasional unyielding individual in your clinical practice who is convinced that hypnosis will open the should-be-sealed portal to his mind for unwanted spirits and demons who are just dying (sorry, pun again intended) to possess his vulnerable soul.

David had a client with a severe case of panic and agoraphobia who expressed ambivalence about hypnosis, preferring to discuss the matter with a church elder before initiating treatment. During his follow-up visit, the middle-aged man told David that his church elder strongly discouraged him from participating in hypnosis, and even went so far as to caution him to be alert while in David's office, as he thought David "might try to put you under when you least expect it." While resisting the urge to laugh out loud, David respected the man's decision, assuring him that he certainly did not want him to participate in anything that made him uncomfortable. However, when informing the man that, during hypnosis, the therapist simply serves as a guide and the client predominantly remains in control of the experience, the client abruptly arose from his chair, and before a frightful exit out of the office, told David, "That's exactly what the elder told me you'd say to try to get me to go under your crazy spell!"

Realize, not everyone will be open and willing to participate in hypnosis. When individuals like the reluctant gentleman in the above scenario cringe in fear at the notion of hypnosis, it is best to leave well enough alone and offer other therapeutic interventions that will be met with greater acceptance. After all, without a certain level of "buy-in" from your clients about your treatment interventions (especially when it comes to hypnosis), your endeavors are likely to lead to frustrating and fruitless results.

In general, however, it has fortunately been our experience that when individuals are reasonably motivated to change unwanted behaviors and are fairly open-minded and relatively trusting, an appropriate introduction to hypnosis, including a brief discussion of the truths and myths of hypnosis, will be eagerly embraced and appreciated. For many, hypnosis is a fascinating topic of discussion. Just leave any text on hypnosis (including this one) lying around and see how long it takes for someone within eyeshot of your book to initiate a conversation on the subject. Whether the person asks you if anyone can be hypnotized, if you can hypnotize her *now*, or if she believes the whole matter to be nothing but a bunch of paranormal hogwash, people are generally fascinated with hypnosis. As such, most people are open to a conversation about hypnosis, especially if they believe it can help them overcome some unwanted behavior, emotion, or fear, or help enhance performance, be it academic, athletic, or sexual.

On that note, we will now venture forth, with the understanding that there is likely to be a wide range of experience and competency with hypnosis among our readers. In this chapter and the following one, we will offer a succinct introduction to hypnosis, including a brief review of its history, of what is scientifically understood (and not) about hypnosis, and of strategies for facilitating and deepening your client's trance experiences and, finally, provide pragmatic strategies that can be readily employed in your work with habit control.

WHAT IS HYPNOSIS?

Hypnosis has no single, agreed-upon definition (Lynne & Rhue, 1991; Yapko, 2003). The Society of Psychological Hypnosis, a division of the American Psychological Association dedicated to the science and practice of hypnosis, offers a widely cited and generalized definition (1993):

> Hypnosis is a procedure during which a health professional or researcher suggests that a client, patient, or subject experience changes in sensations, perceptions, thoughts, or behavior.

This broad definition reasonably depicts the relationship between the person doing the hypnosis, the person receiving the hypnosis, and the context of the process itself. Yet there is so much more to hypnosis than that offered above that a single-sentence definition may never suffice. It is the *process* itself, the mix of the give-and-take among provider, receiver, and context, that generates disagreement among the "experts" in the field, thereby challenging a universal definition of hypnosis.

Hypnosis Invented

So the Lord God caused the man to fall into deep sleep....
                                                       —*Genesis 2:21*

Like most subject matters intriguing the intellectually curious, hypnosis possesses a rich history with engaging, trance-like stories filled with a cast of colorful characters that at times seems more fiction than fact. Referenced in literature, cinema, music, and early medical texts, hypnosis continues to be credited and criticized, rightly and wrongly, for possessing powerful influences over the subconscious mind. Of all the behavioral health subject matters we bring up with our lay friends, hypnosis is the one likely to generate the most engaging conversations. Mention the word "hypnosis" in any benign social context and an inquisition like that at a White House press conference just might unfold: Does it really work? Can most people be hypnotized? Can you really make someone quack like a duck? Yes, yes, and well...yes are the respective answers. More on the quacking later.

Of all the possible questions we are asked about hypnosis, our favorite by far is the one inquiring about its history; or, as David's 8-year-old son once asked, "Who invented hypnosis?"

Imhotep

In one form or another, hypnosis has been practiced throughout recorded history and can be traced back 4,000 years to the ancient Egyptian priest Imhotep, whose name literally means "He comes in peace." Inscriptions on "sleep or dream temple" walls dating to Imotep's time tell stories of miraculous cures produced by Egyptian priests invoking trance-like states to cast out "bad spirits" from the minds and bodies of the sick (Osler, 2004). Though Imhotep existed as a mythological figure in the minds of most scholars until the end of the nineteenth century, he was finally established as a historical person after being recognized as the architect of the Step Pyramid of Djoser, the first structure of its kind in Egypt. More relevant for our discussion, he is also credited with establishing Egyptian medicine and founding a school of medicine 2,200 years before Hippocrates was born. It has also been speculated that Imhotep was one of three possible authors of the Edwin Smith Papyrus, the world's earliest known medical document, identifying more than 90 anatomical terms and 48 traumatic injuries (Grimal, 1988; Lehner, 1997). Thanks in part to Hollywood executives, Imhotep's fictionalized status was resurrected in the title role of the 1932 film classic, *The Mummy,* and reanimated in the 1999 remake of the same name.

Hippocrates (1400 B.C.)

Hippocrates, regarded by many as the father of modern medicine, is credited with being the first person to document a mind–body connection that, as we now know, is the basis of hypnotic interventions. Though offering no direct insight into trance phenomena, Hippocrates' preferred means of treatment, like hypnosis, was passive and involved an appreciation that the human body possessed an innate capacity to heal itself (Garrison, 1966).

Paracelsus (1493–1541 A.D.)

Known in some circles as the father of toxicology and credited with naming the element zinc, Paracelsus pioneered the use of chemicals and minerals in medicine, hypothesizing that the attainment of health involved maintaining a delicate balance of minerals within the body (Debus & Multhauf, 1966). Scoffing at his peers for their failure to recognize and appreciate the healing elements of nature, and openly rejecting the Galenic medicine practice of that time (based on Hippocrates' four bodily humors—blood, yellow bile, black bile, and phlegm), Paracelsus sentenced himself to a nomadic life. Though his critics outnumbered his followers, his steadfast and idiosyncratic perspectives on health, particularly the harmonious relationship between man (the microcosm) and nature (the macrocosm), laid the foundation for the development and utilization of current healing practices, including hypnosis.

Franz Anton Mesmer (1734–1815)

Based in part on Paracelsus' theory that heavenly bodies exerted an influence upon disease and healing, Austrian physician Franz Anton Mesmer investigated a process he identified as "animal magnetism," believing all living creatures possessed a magnetic force within them that was responsible for maintaining and relieving illness. After opening a vein and letting a patient bleed for a while, Mesmer discovered that he could inhibit blood flow by passing a magnet over the wound.

Mesmer's primary influence on hypnosis comes from his radical treatment of patients, initially involving magnets to produce an "artificial tide" that in turn promoted a healing process. Eventually, Mesmer dispensed with the magnets, believing that he himself possessed an abundance of animal magnetism that could ease the disturbed ebb and flow of fluid within a human organism, resulting in remarkable and previously unseen cures.

When we consider his methods for the treatment of mental or nervous illness, it is easy to see how Mesmer has been credited with influencing the practice of hypnosis. While seated before a patient, with his knees touching theirs, he would look fixedly in the individual's eyes, make "passes" with his hands from their shoulders down along the sides of their arms, and then press his fingers on an area just below the individual's diaphragm. At times, Mesmer maintained pressure on the diaphragm for several hours until a convulsion, providing objective evidence that unhealthy obstructions were finally unblocked, was witnessed. Perhaps for some, this description conjures up images of a televangelist releasing some demon-possessed illness afflicting a physically or emotionally pained member of the congregation. Though we don't encourage you to embark upon a study attempting to prove or disprove Mesmer, we maintain that continuous pressure applied to a person's diaphragm for several hours is likely to eventually engender a convulsion, in either the recipient or provider of said pressure!

Following a failed attempt to heal a young blind musician, and group interventions resembling freakish séances, Mesmer's work came under close scrutiny by other orthodox medical practitioners. In 1784, his reputation, and the practice of animal magnetism in particular, were put on the line when King Louis XVI appointed a four-member committee from the Faculty of Medicine to investigate whether Mesmer had indeed discovered a new physical fluid that could be influenced by external sources. Of particular interest to the King was Mesmer's Salon, where he employed a large round oak barrel, or *baquet*, that was used to treat a large group of people. With Mesmer's reputation as a remarkable healer spreading throughout Paris and a demand for his services exceeding his ability to meet it, the *baquet*, like most inventions, became an inevitable creation born of necessity. Essentially, the *baquet* was a large round oak barrel containing vessels of magnetized water, containing iron filings and glass filaments, which enabled a group of people to simultaneously receive treatment by permitting individual access to iron rods that projected from the barrel's cover. With his subjects sitting or standing around the *baquet*, at times holding hands to assist the circulation of the magnetized fluid, Mesmer would move about, talking softly and making passes either with an iron wand or with his hands. Entrancing piano music typically accompanied the procedure; on occasion, Mesmer himself would play a glass armonica to enhance the mood. (For a reconstruction of the ambiance likely established by Mesmer's glass armonica—*not* harmonica—visit http://en.wikipedia.org/wiki/Glass_armonica, where the soothing sounds of this instrument can be heard.)

At the request of the Faculty of Medicine committee, the King appointed five additional commissioners from the Royal Academy of Sciences, comprising distinguished contemporary physicians and academicians, including Antoine-Laurent Lavoisier, Joseph-Ignace Guillotine, and Benjamin Franklin. The commission concluded that Mesmer's so-called "animal magnetism" and "artificial tide" did not exist and proclaimed him to be a deceiver and charlatan whose "healings" were due to the fantasy of his patients. Forced to leave Paris in 1785, Mesmer eventually settled in Switzerland, where he spent most of the last thirty years of his life in seclusion.

Whether remembering him as a charlatan, quack, or physician whose insight into the mind–body connection was ahead of his time, the field of hypnosis owes a small debt of gratitude to the man whose name is now part of our language.

During Mesmer's declining years, his pupil and friend, the Marquis de Puysegur, continued to practice and teach animal magnetism through the expansion of an establishment founded by Mesmer in 1782 called the Society of Harmony. For a substantial fee, subscribers would receive full instruction in Mesmer's methods and an opportunity to practice mesmerism in specified towns. Though we could find no definitive verification of the matter, there are documented reports that Puysegur's student and friend, Professor Jean Deleuze, demonstrated what is likely to be the first incident of posthypnotic suggestion. But it was Baron Dupotet de Sennevoy, animal magnetism practitioner and lecturer, whose influence on another Commission of Enquiry set up by the Academy of Science ultimately vindicated Mesmer and his theory of animal magnetism.

John Elliotson (1791–1868)

Though perhaps better known for introducing the use of the stethoscope and other medical advances in England, John Elliotson became fascinated with the lectures of Dupotet and began his own researches into animal magnetism. In 1843, Elliotson and some of his colleagues founded a quarterly journal called *The Zoist*, to which Elliotson contributed several medical articles, including case studies involving painless mesmeric operations. Though this journal spawned the development of several mesmeric institutions, and much of the literature published within *The Zoist* would be acceptable even by today's publication standards, it couldn't withstand the criticism and ridicule of its detractors for dedicating space to less tolerable, eccentric practices like clairvoyance, phrenology, and odylic force. In December 1855, *The Zoist* was, to put it kindly, laid to rest.

James Esdaile (1808–1859)

Of all the authors published in *The Zoist*, perhaps the most prolific contributor, known for successfully employing mesmeric analgesia in numerous operations, was James Esdaile. Though Esdaile was not the first to use mesmeric analgesia, in 1846 he operated a small hospital in Calcutta and another in 1848 that relied upon mesmerism in thousands of "painless operations," including 19 amputations. Eventually, the introduction of chloroform for painless surgery signaled the virtual end of analgesic mesmerism.

James Braid (1795–1860)

James Braid, a Scottish surgeon of high repute, coined the terms "hypnotism," "hypnotise," and "hypnotic," borrowing from the Greek word for sleep, *hypnos*. Initially a skeptic of the somnambulistic state, Braid became a convert of the controversial séance after forcing a pin beneath a fingernail of a "mesmerized" girl who showed no signs of discomfort. After applying a more rigorous scientific investigation of hypnosis, many influential people began to more readily embrace the technique. Of his many contributions that advanced the practice of hypnosis was his assertion that hypnotic effects involved a subjective phenomenon and were not produced by the hypnotizer, as many of his time believed.

The Nancy School, founded by Auguste Ambrose Liebeault (1823–1904) and Hippolyte Bernheim (1840–1919), offered significant contributions that advanced the acceptance of hypnotherapy, as it provided these men with opportunities to practice hypnosis on their hospitalized patients. Though difficult to confirm with any degree of confidence, it has been reported that Bernheim used hypnotic inductions on about 5,000 patients over the course of four years with a 75% success rate (International Association of Pure Hypnoanalysts, 2007).

Jean Martin Charcot (1835–1893)

In the same year that Bernheim and Leibeault met, 1882, Jean Martin Charcot presented his findings on hypnotism to the French Academy of Sciences. Unlike Bernheim and Leibeault, who maintained that hypnosis was a direct result of suggestion, Charcot concluded that hypnosis was simply a manifestation of hysteria. Most of his conclusions were based on his experience working as a neurologist with 12 hysterical patients at Saltpetriere. Given Charcot's limited pool of subjects, The Nancy School position won out in the end and influenced the continued acceptance and practice of hypnosis.

Sigmund Freud (1856–1939)

In 1885, Sigmund Freud visited Charcot and, after directly observing clinical demonstrations, was so impressed with hypnosis that he translated Bernheim's *De la Suggestion* into German and introduced his friend and colleague Joseph Breuer to the technique. In 1895, he and Breuer published their classic work, *Studies in Hysteria*, which was based in part on their work using hypnosis.

Freud eventually abandoned the practice after a female patient awakened from an induced trance and threw her arms around his neck.

Proffering positive transference—positive feelings toward and attraction to the therapist, including the desire to please him—as the source behind the mystery of hypnosis, Freud wrote, "I was modest enough not to attribute the event to my own irresistible personal attraction, and I felt that I had now grasped the nature of the mysterious element that was at work behind hypnotism."

Pierre Janet (1859–1947)

Pierre Janet was a pioneering French psychiatrist credited with coining the terms *dissociation* and *subconscious*. Janet introduced the concept of dissociation, positing that hysterical symptoms arise from subconscious fixed ideas that have been isolated and usually forgotten, split off from consciousness, and that symbolically embody painful experiences. He studied under Charcot in Paris and, because of his introduction of the concept of automatism, he, rather than Freud, is considered by some to be the true founder of psychoanalysis (Bliss, 1986).

Clark L. Hull (1884–1952)

Clark L. Hull was a very influential American psychologist who is frequently credited with having initiated the modern study of hypnosis. His 1933 work *Hypnosis and Suggestibility* involved 10 years of rigorous study of hypnosis phenomena, applying statistical and experimental analysis that in the end demonstrated that hypnosis had no connection with sleep, as had been proposed by many method skeptics. At the same time, Hull's findings tempered many extravagant claims about hypnosis, including remarkable improvements in cognition or extraordinary sensory capabilities. Through his efforts, with the assistance of 20 research associates, Dr. Hull managed to promote a sense of respectability for hypnosis in the scientific community, thereby setting the stage for subsequent objective evaluation of what over time has become a less controversial subject and more acceptable means of treatment of unwanted behaviors.

Though concerned that his seminal work on hypnosis might stigmatize him in ways that would be less than complimentary, Hull maintained faith and confidence that his work would offer significant contributions to hypnotherapy and the field of psychology in general. In one of his diary entries he wrote, "I believe, however, that the book itself has been worth doing from the point of view of the advancement of science. I believe that it is an important contribution, that it may mark a new epoch in that form of experimentation, and that it will be read and quoted for a long time, possibly a hundred years" (Hull, 1962, p. 852). After 75 years his prediction holds true, as many of Hull's findings concerning hypnosis continue to stand the test of time.

Milton H. Erickson (1901–1980)

Milton H. Erickson is considered by many to be the most innovative and influential figure in the modern practice of hypnosis. In the next chapter, the hypnotherapy techniques discussed, as you will see, are borrowed heavily from Dr. Erickson's teachings and writings, as we have found them to be very effective for our work with helping people eliminate unwanted behaviors.

Dr. Erickson's personal history no doubt influenced the theoretical framework that we understand as strategic hypnosis. Though not a term coined by Erickson, it aptly depicts his creative, well-conceived, and focused strategies aimed at relieving some unwanted symptom. Stricken with polio at age 17, paralyzed and initially unable to move anything other than his eyeballs, Erickson frequently remarked about what a good teacher polio had been, as it forced him to relearn how to move and how to perceive his world. His nearly mythical story is inspirational and is frequently included in David's introduction to hypnosis, as it brings a human element to its techniques and benefits. For an engaging and educational "take" on the foundation of Dr. Erickson's principles of therapy and hypnosis, we encourage you to read *Taproots: Underlying Principles of Milton Erickson's Therapy and Hypnosis* (1987), written by our friend and colleague Bill O'Hanlon. As an aside, Bill who has been very instrumental in the field of brief solution-oriented therapy, worked as Erickson's gardener for a year while absorbing whatever knowledge and experience he could gather to enhance his own clinical work as a therapist.

Unlike his predecessor and mentor, Clark L. Hull, PhD, Erickson dismissed the ritualized, nearly robotic approach to hypnosis and instead recognized and respected individual differences among people, capitalizing on the unique attributes of the person for formulating strategic interventions. Dr. Erickson can also be credited with popularizing a more natural and conversational approach to hypnosis that relied on storytelling, paradox, metaphors, and a belief that people had powerful unconscious resources that could be accessed and mobilized for therapeutic purposes and productive outcomes.

It is impossible to parse out Dr. Erickson's contributions to hypnosis without appreciating his reliance upon nonhypnotic interventions, such as communication dynamics within a family system and other strategic and at times seemingly paradoxical task assignments, including symptom prescription to enhance greater symptom control. We are confident that Erickson and many of his disciples would argue that all therapy, including the above ingredients, involve at least a subtle spicing of hypnosis.

9 Ericksonian Hypnosis

The universe is change; our life is what our thoughts make it.

—Marcus Aurelius Antoninus

In chapter 8, we summarized the relevant contributions of individuals who helped shape the practice of hypnosis as we know it today. Though there have been several important contributors since Milton Erickson's, for the purpose of this book and our work with individuals desiring to permanently change unwanted behavior, we primarily employ the principles and techniques espoused by Dr. Erickson. In this chapter, we will address several key components of Ericksonian hypnosis, including utilization, presupposition, matching, linking, and chaining and how to apply these techniques and strategies in our work with habit control. As in chapter 3, vis à vis Enneagrams, the present chapter offers an overview of Ericksonian hypnosis and is not meant to be an exhaustive exploration of hypnotherapy à la Milton Erickson. Hopefully, however, by the conclusion of this chapter, you will have adequate information to start applying these techniques when working with your clients.

INTRODUCING HYPNOSIS TO YOUR CLIENT

Preparing a client for hypnosis is crucial for enhancing efficacy and in many ways serves as the initial stage of formal induction into trance.

In our collective experience, though most of our clients have been amenable to the idea of hypnosis to help them manage unwanted behaviors, some remain cautious, skeptical, and resistant to the idea of "going under a spell." In essence, the trepidation can be boiled down to a few issues: (a) fear of the unknown, (b) harbored fear for something that should not be frightening, and/or (c) limited faith that hypnosis will be effective in eradicating the behavior of concern. These potential impediments all make sense in light of the exposure many people have encountered at State Fairs and Renaissance Festivals that challenge the face validity of hypnosis by perpetuating the misconception that it largely involves "mind control."

Traditional hypnosis, which is to be distinguished from Ericksonian hypnosis, generally relies on the specific instructions or directives of a therapist, underscoring the need to do as the therapist suggests. Telling clients to "close your eyes" or suggesting "your eyelids **are** getting heavy" or "when I count backwards from 10 to 1, you will be in a deep, relaxing trance" is very directive, controlling, and in some ways presumptuous. If the person is not in deep trance by the time the countdown is done, someone failed to do his job, and usually the onus falls on the client, who is perceived as resistant, unhypnotizable, or just not ready to overcome their behavior(s) of concern.

Ericksonian hypnosis bypasses this element of control by using permissive words that offer clients options or choices that can be individualized and made more suitable for them. There is no forced choice. Rather, permissive words and phrases like "You *could* close your eyes" or "Your eyes *might* just close on their own" are less forceful and more inviting. Most people prefer to be in charge of their destiny, one way or the other, especially when they are in an office, sitting or lying in a vulnerable position with their eyes closed!

Additionally, by using what clients bring to the session, we invoke a sense of respect for their own ability to go into trance without invoking much direction or control. Erickson referred to this as the "Utilization Approach" and it involves simply letting clients know that whatever they are doing is fine and as a therapist you can help them use that for enabling trance (Erickson & Rossi, 1979). David (co-author David B. Reid, PsyD) tells his clients frequently that they will find their own way of going into trance, as their unconscious mind knows the best way to do it. Some people fidget, others shake their legs, some laugh, and some sigh. By simply responding to the overt behavior and permitting it within the session, that which might seem to distract from trance can be used to enhance trance. Children at times laugh or fidget during the initial stages of trance work, so we tell them, "Laughing is a great way to go into trance. It's fun, relaxing, and helps the body get in touch with positive energy." Rather than tell a client to "sit perfectly still" or "try not to move so much," we suggest that, "Moving like that can be very helpful for finding the most comfortable way of going into trance. It's your body's way of letting the energy out so that a sense of calm and peace can be created."

Though easing a client's anticipatory anxiety by addressing any myths and misconceptions about hypnosis is important and should not be neglected, making a number of relevant assumptions about hypnosis during the initial session establishes a mind-set of success that can be quite powerful. Erickson referred to this as "presupposition" and relied upon it not only before and during trance, but afterwards as well.

When something is presupposed, there is an assumption that it will and should happen. As with most things anticipated, we can presuppose that something *will* happen, that something *is* happening, and that something *has* just happened. For instance, asking someone if she is going to walk to work, ride the bus to work, or drive to work *presupposes* that the individual will be going to work one way or the other. When David encounters resistance from his teenage children about initiating their homework, rather than argue the matter with them, at times he will ask, "Are you going to do your homework in the kitchen, in the dining room, or in your bedroom?" This question may then be followed with "When you finish your homework do you want to go out and play, watch some television, or eat a snack?" The first question presupposes that the homework will be initiated, the second that it will be completed. The same presupposition principles can be employed when asking clients whether they prefer to go into trance on the couch or in the chair, or while sitting or lying down. We can then presuppose that the trance will have occurred and can end by asking their intentions for the day *after* trance. Additionally, as Erickson was fond of doing, upon the conclusion of a session, we welcome our clients back to the more alert and conscious *waking* world, making the assuming that a trance state did indeed occur.

If you carefully review the above paragraph you will notice we use the word *when* not *if* when presuming that something will happen. Using the word "if" leaves room for doubt, for a potential "failed" experience, whereas the word "when" assumes that something will happen. Table 9.1 offers a number of examples of using presupposition in hypnosis.

When using hypnosis with our clients, it is important to keep in mind that Ericksonian hypnosis is not so much about offering directives (the outside-in approach) as it is about evoking some response from the client (the inside-out approach). Though a narrow definition of hypnosis, the inside-out notion was captured well by Erickson's student, Bill O'Hanlon, who defined trance as "the evocation of involuntary experience" (O'Hanlon & Martin, 1992, p. 11).

Erickson had tremendous faith in people's natural abilities to go into trance and create trance phenomena (Erickson, 1983, 1985; Erickson & Rossi, 1979; Erickson, Rossi, & Rossi, 1976). He would remind his clients of spontaneous and casual trance experiences like losing track of time (disorientation in time), or forgetting why they came into a room (amnesia), or times when they became so distracted or so captivated by something that the experience of physical discomfort/pain was no longer appreciated (anesthesia/analgesia), or when they engaged in automatic behavior without conscious awareness (dissociation), or forgot for a moment where they were (disorientation in place).

Perhaps a personal story will bring this all to life:

> David's brother-in-law Ted walked into a music store to purchase a reed for his saxophone. As the clerk went to the stockroom to retrieve the reed, Ted became distracted by a friend who was walking across the parking lot and heading to a coffee shop. Knowing the clerk would hold the reed for him, Ted walked outside, greeted his friend and engaged in small-talk conversation for a few minutes. After bidding his friend farewell, Ted resumed his shopping, and walked up to the service desk and asked the attendant standing before him about a reed for his sax. The store clerk offered an odd and confused facial gesture which begged Ted to repeat himself. The confused clerk, not knowing quite what to make of his customer's request, kindly said, "This is Radio Shack, we don't sell reeds for saxophones." Ted had unknowingly walked into the wrong store, assumed he was in the music store and failed to take conscious note of all of the Radio Shack signs, including the one on the clerk's nametag until he was properly oriented. As if magically transported to a new place and time, Ted suddenly became abundantly aware of every red and white Radio Shack sign that surrounded him.

Surely you have your own experiences or have witnessed or heard of others' "day-trance" experiences. Keeping track of such experiences

Table 9.1

USING PRESUPPOSITION IN HYPNOSIS*

The following are a number of examples of using presupposition in hypnosis:

1. Give two or more options that lead in the desired direction:
   - Would you like to go into trance now or later?
   - I don't know if you'd like to close your eyes to go into a trance or if you'll keep your eyes open.
   - Would you like to use the recliner or stay where you're seated to go into a trance?

2. Presume that something is about to happen:
   - Before you go into trance, there are some myths about hypnosis that I'd like to dispel.
   - Have you ever been in trance before?
   - When you're in trance, you can do something nice for yourself.
   - Don't go into trance too quickly.

3. Presume that something is happening:
   - You can go deeper.
   - That's right, just continuing.
   - As your unconscious mind continues to help you do what you need to do....

4. Presume that something just happened:
   - How was that?
   - Welcome back!
   - How did that trance compare with the last one?

5. Imply that something is happening, will happen, or has just happened by talking about its rate of occurrence:
   - Don't go in too quickly.
   - I don't know when your unconscious will solve that for you.

6. Imply that something is happening, will happen, or has just happened and wonder aloud whether that person is aware of that:
   - I don't know whether you have noticed that your breathing has changed.
   - You probably aren't aware that your unconscious mind is doing a lot of work for you.

*Reproduced with permission of Bill O'Hanlon (O'Hanlon & Martin, 1992).

and sharing them with your clients helps address the myths of hypnosis and minimizes resistance to a very natural and human phenomenon that all of us experience several times a day. Indeed, if there is anything frightening about trance, it is that many trance experiences occur while people are operating heavy machinery at speeds exceeding the legal limit!

Once a client has consented to treatment, formal trance induction can proceed. At this time, a step-by-step approach to hypnosis may seem the most economical and user-friendly way to learn how to employ hypnosis in your clinical approach. But, like psychotherapy itself, hypnosis involves interactive relations between two or more people that is more complex and cannot be reduced to a concrete flowchart. Appreciating the uniqueness of each person when applying hypnotic strategies is essential if the work is to be beneficial.

A number of assumptions can be inferred from this statement that should not be ignored when doing trance work. First, it is important to recognize that each person has a unique history that he brings into the therapy session which makes him unlike anyone else. Second, this underscores Erickson's method of utilization mentioned above and underscores another assumption that each person will have his own unique way of going into and experiencing trance. Finally, a third assumption concerns the multidimensionality of hypnotic experiences. Hypnosis will inevitably involve physical, emotional, cognitive, behavioral, and even spiritual features. Each individual may have his own preferred way of enhancing focused attention and experiencing any of the above during trance. The reader is again referred to Yapko's book, *Trancework* (Yapko, 2003), for a more detailed discussion on the phenomenology of hypnotic experiences.

Hypnosis, like therapy, is an art form that becomes manifest based on flexible communication (e.g., verbal and nonverbal) between therapist and client. Nonetheless, there are important techniques that when employed properly enhance the potential benefits of the therapeutic intervention we call hypnosis or trance.

Contextual Cues

Nearly everywhere we go, there are contextual cues providing visceral feedback to our senses. Generally, these contextual cues, whether visual, auditory, tactile, or olfactory, are specific to the setting or circumstances of our individual lives. For instance, if you hear a group of people singing "Happy Birthday" you can safely assume that someone is celebrating a birthday. Walk into any place of worship and you will be immediately greeted with visual (stained-glass windows, pews, religious relics and symbols) and auditory (silence, organ music, choirs singing) stimuli. Because these contextual cues have been repeatedly paired with personal experiences over time, automatic behaviors tend to be elicited. In essence, our reactions to these experiences have been conditioned, much like Pavlov's dogs were conditioned to drool to the sound of a bell.

By taking advantage of classical conditioning principles, we can repeatedly pair specific contextual cues with trance experiences. Eventually, these contextual cues (previously unconditioned and now conditioned stimuli) elicit trance (previously an unconditioned and now a conditioned response). Turning off one's cell phone in and of itself is not initially a cue that hypnosis is about to begin, until it is introduced as such or repeatedly paired with hypnosis. Over time, contextual cues are introduced that "set the mood" and essentially announce that hypnosis is about to begin.

Changing the tone, volume, and rate of your voice, dimming the lights in your office, and moving to a different chair mark behavioral and contextual cues that distinguish "this *is trance*" from "this is *not trance*." At times, we include soft, melodic background music or the subtle sound of a white-noise maker with our hypnosis sessions, but these ambiance creators are generally individualized, as some clients prefer music and others require silence. Observing your client's breathing will allow you to establish a hypnotic rhythm by *speaking on the exhale*. Simply stated, when the client exhales, you speak, when she inhales, you remain silent. When we discuss hand and arm levitation below, you will see how this rhythm can be capitalized upon to evoke a desired response from your client.

Matching

Matching is joining your language behavior and body behavior to your client's language behavior and body behavior. In their text on the techniques of Ericksonian hypnosis, Bandler and Grinder (1975) distinguish between mirroring and cross-mirroring. Mirroring is when you replicate or mime the same body movements, positions, posture, and breathing rate of another person. When they move, you move; when they breathe, you breathe; when they slouch, you slouch, and so on. You match the person's behavior exactly. We should caution you at this point, though, mirroring should be done in very subtle ways because too much mirroring can be unnerving and even irritating.

Another kind of matching is called cross-mirroring, and is the one we usually incorporate during our sessions with our clients, as it is less obvious and tends to promote the kind of response we are seeking from our client. Unlike mirroring per se, where behavior is mimed, cross-mirroring involves co-varying the behaviors of another person. Cross-mirroring is particularly effective for helping people calm down or relax. For instance, if an agitated individual is flailing his hands and arms in exaggerated manners while raising his voice, we could cross-mirror this behavior with a nod of the head each time the person exhales, or every time his body moves to one side or shifts position in the chair, we may raise our hand slightly. As we match the person's behavior, we can slow our responses down or adjust our behavior like slowing down our breathing in an effort to get him to shift his behavior to match ours, which is slower, calmer, more settled. Those of us who have done crisis work appreciate the importance of matching a hostile individual's loud, pressured speech with a lower, calmer, slower rhythm and rate.

Descriptive Matching

Descriptive matching, to paraphrase Detective Jack Webb of *Dragnet* fame, involves the facts, and just the facts. Bill O'Hanlon likens it to a radio commentator describing the action in the "sport of hypnosis to the folks at home with their ears to the radio" (O'Hanlon & Martin, 1992, p. 26). With descriptive matching you don't go beyond that which you can see and hear. There are no inferences (nor assumptions) about internal feeling states. Though it is tempting to make statements like "You're sitting there, comfortable and relaxed," this is an assumption. Though the person may look comfortable and relaxed, internally they may be experiencing some level of discomfort and your comment would be off-base. Saying "You're sitting there, hands on your lap, feet on the floor...eyes closed" states only facts.

Think of descriptive matching as a human biofeedback machine. It simply involves relaying that which you can see and hear and would be affirmed by your client. This lends credibility to what you are doing as you are reporting the plain truth and not going beyond that which is actually happening and can be verified. Descriptive matching also helps your client narrow the focus of her attention. Trance involves a narrowing of focused attention that ultimately elicits an automatic response from the client. When we describe that which we see, it allows our client to tend to that body part or that experience to the exclusion of other stimuli or distractions.

DOING TRANCEWORK

Once you perceive that your client is in or nearing a trance state (slower breathing, relaxed facial muscles, spontaneous movements, hand and arm levitation) hypnotic interventions can be employed to deepen a trance or address symptoms of concern. Erickson identified a number of therapeutic strategies that have been shown to enhance therapeutic outcome. These include linking, interspersal, splitting, and of course other strategies mentioned above like presupposition and utilization.

Linking

Linking involves joining two things together that have not previously been linked together. Like matching, linking can be verbal or nonverbal and is used to enhance a learning experience as well as enhance trance.

Verbal linking can be evidenced by use of conjunctions like the word "and." For instance you could say, "You are sitting in the chair *and* you can go into a trance." Though sitting in a chair has nothing inherently to do with trance, putting them together makes a stronger association between the two experiences. You could even extend or add to it by saying, "You are sitting in the chair with your eyes closed, your breathing gently slowing, *and* you can go into trance."

Contingent linking can be a bit stronger because it makes a more direct implication. Words like "as," "when," and "where" offer contingent linking experiences: "As you sit in that chair, listening to my voice, you can go into trance" or "When you sit there, all the way down in the chair, you can go into trance."

Linking, like permissiveness and presupposition, can also be used to connect an individual's experience to the understanding that he can (and will) go into trance. It offers a win–win predicament, so that no matter what the client does or experiences, it can be used in ways to promote and enhance trance. Words like "more" or "less" offer the link. In *Solution Oriented Hypnosis*, Bill O'Hanlon identifies four kinds of linking that can involve the "more or less" terminology: "The more this, the more that" or "the less this, the less that" or "the more this, the less that" or "the less this, the more that." For instance, if someone seems to be distracted by extraneous stimuli, you could suggest, "The more your conscious mind is distracted by sounds outside this room, the easier it can be for your unconscious mind to help you go into trance as it can be freed from the control of your conscious mind." In essence the suggestion is: the more distracted you are the easier it is to go into trance. The same method can be applied to someone who seems restless and is having difficulty settling into a comfortable position. Children are typically very squirmy and offering them a link that "the more you move around, the easier it will be for you to become comfortable and go into trance" can be helpful.

The above examples imply a linkage between experiences that are happening at the same time and are used to help promote trance. Another kind of linking can be used to enhance trance and promote a learning experience. It is called *causal* linking and involves a cause-and-effect relationship in which you claim that something causes or will cause something to occur. Making the inference that "a comfortable trance will allow your unconscious mind to be more available and mobilize and access resources in creative ways" is one such example. This form of linking should be used sparingly as it implies more of a coerced suggestion that transfers more control of the trance work to the therapist.

We also use linking to promote permanent habit control. Suggesting that "the heavier that arm feels, the deeper your trance can be, and the stronger your resistance to lighting up a cigarette/eating that piece of cake or candy bar." Or we can link the current hypnotic trance to some future experience: "The lighter your hand and arm can feel, the more your unconscious mind is able to help you stay focused on your goals of becoming a permanent nonsmoker (or) of experiencing the ideal body you want to have."

Finally, you can link the client's current hypnotic experience to past common everyday trance experiences, as mentioned above. Telling a story about your own trance experiences or offering opportunities for your client to recall some of her own trance states can be helpful for minimizing resistance and promoting a here-and-now trance that is nonthreatening.

Splitting

Splitting is almost the opposite of linking. Splitting involves separating into parts something that is perceived as a unified entity. The most common kind of split that occurs in hypnosis is one that occurs between the conscious mind and the unconscious mind. In this particular case, of course, the split is a linguistic one, since this is not a distinction that occurs in the real world. Despite the universal recognition of these terms, neuroscientists have yet to locate the neurological underpinnings of either the conscious or unconscious mind.

During hypnosis work, to help a client go into trance, stay in trance, or deepen the trance, we can create verbal and nonverbal splits between the conscious and unconscious mind. Though mentioning the distinction between the two, you can lean in one direction when mentioning the conscious mind (right side) and another when mentioning the unconscious mind (left side). Whether the client's eyes are open or shut, the distinction, or split, can still be made as, in either case, your voice is cast in one of two directions. To make an even clearer distinction, we vary our voice tone depending on which part of the mind we are speaking about.

When introducing the split between the conscious (**louder** voice tone) and unconscious (*softer* voice tone) mind, we may say the following:

Consciously (lean right) **you may not really understand what it is like to go into trance,** *while unconsciously* (lean left) *your mind probably has lots of experience with going into trance.* So, **you could be sitting there now, consciously** (lean right) **wondering if you can really go into trance,** *and unconsciously* (lean left) *your mind may already be helping you go into trance, just like it does spontaneously like when you stare into a fire or listen to the ocean.*

The above example shows how you can split between the conscious and unconscious minds and do so both verbally and nonverbally. To generate an even greater impact, with practice you can begin to use different facial expressions when splitting the conscious and unconscious minds. In a way, this begins to foster descriptive matching that, over time, if used repeatedly with your clients, will serve to facilitate or promote trance.

Similarly, we can split between the here-and-now present (external focus) to the then-and-there past or future (internal focus). By redirecting a person's focus away from the here-and-now (i.e., away from the descriptive matching mentioned above) to then-and-there, which can be any place other than here, at any time other than now (i.e., past or future), we help direct a person's focus away from the current life problem(s) that confront this person to a time in the future (or past) when the problem is not (or was not) present. We have found this to be particularly beneficial in our work with people who desire to quit smoking or acquire their ideal body, as we can go to a time in the past when the person did not smoke or when he weighed less, or take the person to the future where he will not smoke or will acquire the body he desires.

As we guide people into trance, we help them focus internally on the then-and-there, and once trance is near complete, we help them focus on a more external, here-and-now experience by changing the tone of our voice to match the "conscious voice" mentioned before and reminding them of where they are (e.g., sitting in the chair, arms by your sides, feet on the floor) while preparing them to slowly open their eyes so they can become accustomed to the lighting in the room.

Interspersal

Some would say that interspersal is a more advanced technique that involves the combination of both linking and splitting. With interspersal, we repeatedly mark out certain words or phrases within the context of a hypnosis session. Interspersal can be used to deepen the hypnotic experience, to facilitate the experience of a specific hypnotic phenomenon, to "implant" ideas for future reference, or to simply reiterate some important point or lesson (Erickson, 1966).

David frequently uses interspersal during an individual's first formal hypnosis experience because it seems very effective for helping people experience trance. It can also be very effective when the message being interspersed within the session is timed with the client's breathing. For instance in the below example, imagine that each time an italicized word is spoken, it is timed with the client's exhale:

> With your eyes closed, your arms resting there on your lap [descriptive matching], just take a slow *deep* breath if you'd like and slowly release. And you can do that two, or three, or more times if you like so each *deep* breath coming from *deep* within your body can release any sense of tension or stress. And when you're ready, if you'd like [a suggestion, not demand], just imagine that you are sitting by a poolside, just observing, watching. And as you sit there, perhaps *deep* in *thought*, you notice different people going into the pool. You notice that each one goes *into* the pool differently. One person walks slowly up to the pool and *goes in* one step at a time. Gradually...slowly...waiting...letting his body get used to the water before he *goes in* any *deeper*. He takes a few more steps...stops and waits, the water now up to his knees. After a few more seconds, he decides to *go in a little farther...deeper*. And may eventually *go all the way in* or may wait and not *go all the way in* [notice the distinction after the word "not"]. At the same time, you may notice another person sitting on the side of the pool. Her legs are dangling in the water. Though her body is not *all the way in,* her legs are in the water. And she may just stay there or she may decide to slowly *go all the way in.* Maybe eventually she decides to *go in deeper.* And then there are other people who you see there at the pool who walk up to the side of the pool and maybe dip their toes in the water before they just dive *all the way in.* And those are just some ways people can go into a pool. And these are ways that you can *go into trance.* You can *go into trance* slowly, methodically, one step at a time before you decide to *go deeper.* Or like the person sitting on the side of the pool, you can go part-way *into trance* so that maybe only part of you is *in trance* and another part of you, maybe consciously isn't *in trance.* And I even know some people who are very familiar with *going into trance* and can come into my office and just like the person diving *all the way into* the pool can just sit down there where you are, close their eyes, and within a matter of a minute can *go into trance.*

As you can see from examining the italicized words above, we have interspersed and emphasized certain words that facilitate trance and help foster a deeper trance. Erickson was known for not only interspersing words by emphasizing his tone of voice, volume, or rate of speech, but for touching his clients' arm when saying certain words. Of course if you plan to do this, be sure to forewarn your client before initiating formal hypnosis and ensure that she has consented to being touched.

For us, it is a rare occurrence when we touch our clients, though at times, using touch can be clinically relevant and helpful (e.g., patients with pain disorders or other somatic illnesses).

With skeptical clients, interspersal can be helpful for facilitating the trance experience that they doubt will occur. For instance you can doubt along with your client about the possibility of initiating trance and doing so while interspersing certain words:

> I'm not really sure if you consciously believe that you can *go into trance,* and I really don't know how *deeply* you may or may not *go into a trance.* Some people just need time to *go into trance* and maybe the conscious mind has a hard time with *letting go* to allow the unconscious mind the opportunity to *go into trance.*

A GLOBAL POSITIONING SYSTEM FOR HYPNOSIS*

The global positioning system (GPS) is a welcome device when traveling in unfamiliar territory. It offers a sense of comfort and security, knowing that you are unlikely to get lost, and even if you do, this handy instrument will guide you back on course so that you reach your ultimate destination. Though we can't offer "real time" directions for hypnosis, we can at least provide the following guidelines to ensure that you stay on track and also provide you with some redirection suggestions should you feel "lost."

The first thing we should tell you before embarking on our step-by-step enhance-the-trance list is to *BREATHE.* As simple and condescending as it sounds, the one thing that we have observed novice hypnotherapists do is hold their breath or breathe irregularly thereby throwing their timing and rhythm off.

As David Bader notes in his satirical pocket book *Zen Judaism: For You a Little Enlightenment* (2002): Breathe in, breathe out, breathe in, breathe out. Forget this and attaining enlightenment will be the least of your concerns.

Setting the stage, we believe, is frequently neglected or overlooked by many therapists. Preparing a client for hypnosis serves as a solid

---

*Inspired by Bill O'Hanlon's "The Hitchhiker's Guide to Hypnosis" from *Solution Oriented Hypnosis* (O'Hanlon & Martin, 1992).

foundation for a successful hypnosis experience. For us, there are two primary components of hypnosis work. It is important to note that we are not simply providing the client with information, but we are actually initiating the hypnotic process. When David learns a new *kata* in his Kempo Karate class, it is almost assured that for the first several weeks he will look like an intoxicated kangaroo on roller blades. Over time, after a little dose of public humiliation (and support) the *kata* becomes second-hand, automatic, internalized, as "muscle memory" takes over and the form becomes effortless, fluid, and rhythmic.

Your first hypnosis session with your willing client may be a bit awkward, intimidating, and may perhaps feel contrived. We suggest you tell your client that this is a new skill you are learning though it can still be beneficial to her. We also suggest you select a client with whom you have a solid therapeutic relationship, as this client will be far more forgiving of any "hiccups" you may experience. The client may also be far more likely to experience the benefits of hypnosis as the trust barrier has already been overcome and, one hopes, the client will be far more comfortable being in an office with you with eyes closed, sitting or lying in a rather vulnerable position. Never underestimate the amount of trust that is required of a client willing to engage in hypnosis.

Unlike most therapeutic tasks or interventions you may have learned in graduate school or during postdoctoral fellowships, hypnosis can be "practiced" on any willing friends or family members. For our colleagues familiar with psychological or neuropsychological testing, you may recall that family members and friends were initial guinea pigs when learning the procedures of a new test. So, breathe in, breathe out, snag a loved one and have fun.

Step 1: Ease Into Things and Start Wherever Your Client Is

If the client is nervous, validate this for him. Give the client permission to think, feel, experience whatever it is he is experiencing. We typically suggest that the person get "as comfortable" as he can. Realize this doesn't mean completely and utterly at ease or relaxed, it simply means what we said, "as comfortable as he can be."

> SUGGESTION: "Just be as comfortable as you can be. Whatever that means for you is fine. If it means you'll be more comfortable going into

trance sitting there, that's fine. If you'd be more comfortable lying down, that's fine too. Whatever works for you. You can even change your mind at any time if you think you'd be more comfortable in some other position."

If the client seems to be resisting trance, whether consciously or unconsciously, validate the experience, make it part of the process of trance, and assure the individual that what she is doing is fine. Usually this happens with people who start laughing or smiling nervously.

> SUGGESTION: "That's right, you can find your own special way into trance. Laughing [moving, stretching, fidgeting, whatever he is doing] is a great way to go into trance. Your mind and body know just what to do to help you go into trance."

Step 2: Find Your Rhythm

Don't forget to breathe! Notice how your client is breathing, speak on their exhale. Skipping a few breaths is fine as long as you maintain a rhythm of speaking when your client exhales. Add a few "go into trance" suggestions as the client exhales. Sometimes, we like to gently rock back and forth to establish a steady rhythm with our client's breathing. You will find that as you do this your movements and her breathing will eventually slow (a sure sign of trance).

Step 3: Expect Success

Presume that the person will go into trance and will obtain the intended results.

> SUGGESTION: "I don't know how quickly or deeply you will go into trance. You will discover that yourself. Maybe even now you notice how you feel different from when you first came in and sat down. Maybe you can even notice that one part of your body is very comfortable and more relaxed and can help the rest of you go into trance."

Step 4: Suggest Automatic Changes

As best as we can understand, trance works well when automatic changes in behavior are suggested and then evidenced. This helps establish a dissociation between the conscious and unconscious mind. After all, if the change is "automatic" and not under the operation of the conscious mind, it therefore by default must be under the control of the unconscious mind. Witnessing these changes as therapists also allows us the opportunity to gauge just where the client is in trance and whether or not other deepening techniques are necessary. In essence, it operates as a feedback system for the client and therapist.

> SUGGESTION: "Your hands can become heavier and heavier with each breath you exhale. Maybe one feels heavier than the other. One may be lighter. So light that that hand can begin to lift up. Getting lighter and lighter as the other hand becomes heavier. You don't even have to think about it because that lighter hand can feel like there isn't anything beneath it at all."

Step 5: Enhance the Trance and Connect It to the Goal

[handwritten annotations: then HOW! what who where why-coping then + now]

Connecting the hypnotic experience to the goal offers additional assistance and strategies that are not otherwise available when conducting more "conscious-oriented" therapy. This process also helps facilitate change as the unconscious mind begins to make or enhance connections that foster healthier choices and minimize self-defeating behavior like overeating or smoking.

> SUGGESTION: "As that hand gets heavier/lighter you can go into trance even deeper, relaxing even more."

> SUGGESTION: "Just like that, as automatic as that, you can see yourself doing things, automatically. Deciding not to smoke that cigarette, knowing and feeling that you don't want it. Just like that your body can automatically do something else instead. Something that is good for you. Something that makes you as comfortable and relaxed as you may be right now."

Step 6: Speak to the Unconscious Mind

This is the essence of hypnosis work. Offering suggestions, direct and indirect, telling stories, using interspersal, anecdotes, and metaphors all speak to the unconscious mind. Understanding that the unconscious mind is very good at controlling and managing automatic processes (e.g., breathing, digesting, heart rate, over-learned motor skills), any behavioral concern (e.g., habit) that appears beyond the conscious control of an individual can benefit from hypnosis. Trance, through the unconscious mind, evokes experiences that can serve as resources and skills to manage unwanted behavior.

> SUGGESTION: When working with an individual who wants to become a permanent nonsmoker we can offer the following: "Your conscious mind knows all the parts of your body. Your arms, legs, lungs, heart. Your unconscious mind knows how to control and manage them. It knows how to move automatically, how to breathe, how to relax. It knows what it needs to do to keep you healthy and well. It even knows how to help make decisions. Knowing these decisions, your unconscious mind can help you become a permanent nonsmoker. Breathing now, notice how comfortable that feels. How different you feel now. That breathing, controlled by your unconscious mind, knows the kind of breathing that is good for you. Healthy for you."

Step 7: Give Them Control

At some point in the session, preferably after you have witnessed evidence that your client is in a comfortable trance, turn the reigns over to her. Let the client guide the process. This allows her o appreciate how she can access and mobilize resources and in turn minimizes reliance upon the therapist for doing so.

> SUGGESTION: "If it feels right for you, take the time now to find a comfortable place. A place perhaps you know and are familiar with, or a place you create on your own. As you settle in, notice how well you can see and image this place. Colors, shapes, contour of objects can become vivid. Notice what you see, what you feel, what you hear. Maybe you can hear things up close and even in the distance."

This experience allows your client the opportunity to heighten and focus his attention, bringing the unconscious mind into the session.

Step 8: Conclude the Session

We like to conclude our hypnosis sessions with our clients by suggesting they "take" the experience with them and then offer suggestions for future positive results.

SUGGESTION: "You can keep feeling what you're feeling, thinking what you're thinking. Before we bring this all to a close, take a moment and image how you can take this experience with you. How you can make it part of you just like any positive experience you have can become part of you. Whether you imagine all of it can be absorbed and internalized or put in a file somewhere in your mind, you can know it is there for your unconscious mind to access when it needs it later. Just do that and when you believe you have successfully internalized this experience so that it stays with you, begin to become more alert and aware of being here in this room."

Before inviting them to become more alert by stretching or moving about and opening their eyes, we offer them one more suggestion for future benefit.

SUGGESTION: "When you're ready, at your own pace and comfort level, gently come out of trance and become more alert, bringing with you all the resources and abilities you need for helping you now…and later."

If you prefer, you can become more specific, tying their trance experience to their goal. For example, you could say,

SUGGESTION: "When you're ready, at your own pace and comfort level, gently come out of trance, becoming more alert and oriented. Bringing with you all the resources and abilities you need to become a permanent nonsmoker/permanently fit and trim, having the ideal body you desire."

Detours: Silence Is Golden

At times, you may become lost in your own trance while helping someone else with theirs. You may lose focus, not know where to go or what to say. Like a novelist with writer's block, you are a hypnotherapist with trance block. At times like this, silence is truly golden. You can use it to your advantage to regroup, brainstorm, and assist your client.

SUGGESTION: "Just continue to feel comfortable. That's right. Maybe you can become even more comfortable. To help you with that, I'm going to give you a couple of minutes of clock time to see how much more comfortable you can be. I will be quiet for 2 minutes and when I start talking again, you can continue to be comfortable in your trance."

Detours: Unexpected Roadblocks

1. Extraneous noise/distractions: Sometimes, noises, people talking, or other extraneous distractions impede a level of comfort conducive to hypnosis. First, we suggest you do all you can to minimize these experiences. If you work in an office where you share space with others, we suggest you use some visual cue alerting others to the work you are doing. For instance, David puts a miniature orange safety cone outside of his office door to alert anyone in the hallway that a hypnosis session is underway. "Do Not Disturb" signs can also be helpful, but they are not as noticeable as the orange safety cone.

2. Escape: Offer an escape hatch for your client, just in case she is not comfortable or is feeling the need to terminate the session. At any time, though preferably during the earlier portion of trance, you can let your client know that she is in control and is free to discontinue the session if she needs to. This allows the client to maintain a greater sense of control and permits a greater level of trust with you, the therapist. We find this particularly effective with hesitant or guarded clients.

SUGGESTION: "As you continue to be even more comfortable, going even deeper in trance, realize that you are in control of the kind of trance you want. You can go even *deeper* if you want, or, to see how well you can control your trance, go *lighter*. Just experience trance anyway you want. You can even stop it if you need to because you are the one who is really in control. Anytime you want, for whatever reason, you can gradually allow yourself to come out of trance."

3. Sleep: Though never the goal of hypnosis, sometimes clients become so comfortable with the trance that they go in a bit too deep and fall asleep. This is a very real possibility, though easily remedied. It is not too difficult to recognize when a client is about to fall asleep, as his breathing becomes heavier, steadier, and usually can be readily spotted as the jaw drops and "mouth breathing" commences. When you noticed that your client either is asleep or about to fall asleep, simply change the tone and volume of your voice to mimic the voice that you use to help people come out of trance. You may need to speak a little louder but do so in a way that won't startle your client. Below we offer a number of suggestions that you can readily implement when someone falls asleep.

SUGGESTION: "You're doing great, but make sure you stay with me, stay awake. Let your subconscious mind be more alert and available. I know it feels very comfortable right now, but I'm going to speak a little louder so you can stay with me and stay awake."

Sometimes, it may be necessary to touch your client to ensure that she awakens and is able to continue with trance. Under these circumstance, rare as they tend to be, let your client know that you are about to touch her, tap the person gently on the hand or arm until you begin to see evidence that she is no longer sleeping. The above suggestion can then be offered as you keep your voice louder and less soothing.

If you ever use touch with hypnosis, we highly recommend that you inform your clients prior to the trance work that you will be touching them during the session and provide the rational for this plan. Though used judiciously, we have both found touch to be helpful and very therapeutic. Touch can be utilized to reinforce and enhance certain trance experiences. For instance, you can suggest that a person's resolve to not smoke, or his ability to more clearly see himself in the ideal body he desires, can become stronger and more vivid after each time you touch his hand. The association between tactile stimulation and visual imagery can be quite useful for taking the trance to the next level. We should caution, however, that this induction technique should be reserved for clients who have experience with trance or are very comfortable working with you. Direct physical contact like touch in any therapeutic encounter (e.g., hugs, a consoling arm draped across a shoulder) can be very powerful, especially when used in the most respect-ful manner.

HYPNOSIS AND HABIT CONTROL

As you become more familiar and comfortable with using hypnosis, you will find it easier to incorporate suggestions and hypnotic interventions into your sessions with your clients.

Bill O'Hanlon offers a simple and pragmatic model for generating interventions during trance. Calling it the "Class of Problems/Class of Solutions" (see Figure 9.1), O'Hanlon designed this model after making sense of the apparently nonsensical interventions of Milton Erickson. Recognizing that Erickson didn't implement interventions in a straightforward manner, but instead utilized strategies that elicited something from the client that offered solutions to their problems, O'Hanlon appreciated that essentially Erickson was thinking in terms of descriptions, evocation, and analogy. In other words, Erickson would generate a description of the problem, what was involved with doing or *creating* the problem. Rather than consider *why* the person was doing something, he would focus on *how* the person was creating the problem. For instance, if someone was experiencing panic attacks or bedwetting, he would consider what it takes to *make* a panic attack or *how* the person might be doing bedwetting. After describing the problem and how it is created, the next step involves identifying and then evoking resources or a pattern of experience that could address the identified problem. One can evoke resources in many ways therapeutically, though in this case we are doing so through trance.

Using the panic attack scenario, we may consider just *how* a person makes a panic attack. We would perhaps consider how the person is internalizing emotions, how she is initiating a fight-or-flight reaction, how she is creating adrenaline and cortisol to make the heart race faster and turn off the parasympathetic nervous system while turning on the sympathetic nervous system. In this case, the problem is a panic attack and the class of problems is an uncontrolled fight-or-flight phenomenon. The way to control fight-or-flight (or minimize the impact of the sympathetic nervous system) is by enhancing the parasympathetic system response, which is accomplished through rest and relaxation. Panic is essentially the result of the autonomic nervous system gone awry. Through trance, suggestions that facilitate and elicit a relaxation response automatically versus those that are under conscious control, will have a greater impact, as panic attacks, when they occur, are beyond

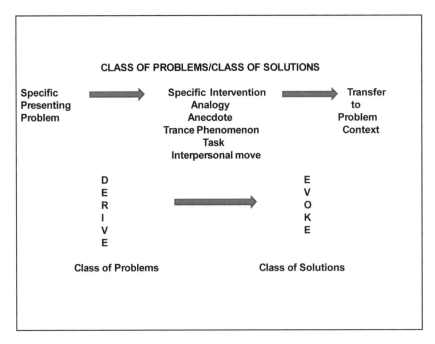

Figure 9.1 Class of problems/class of solutions (reproduced with permission of Bill O'Hanlon).

conscious control. As we mentioned earlier, trance works best for concerns that are involuntary.

With smoking cessation and weight management, the following behavioral issues tend to be beyond conscious control and could directly benefit from hypnosis:

- Smoking cessation:
    - Nicotine withdrawal
    - Chain smoking (automatic behavior of lighting one cigarette with another)
    - Physical reaction preceding smoking (e.g., stress, anxiety)
    - Associations between certain behaviors and cigarettes (e.g. coffee, driving, reading)
- Weight management:

- Binge eating
- Physical stress/anxiety
- Subconscious negative self-statements
- Triggers that promote unhealthy eating habits (ads, images, fast-food restaurants)

Generating a Hypnotic Blueprint for Change

Athletes call it getting "in the zone." Musicians talk about being "in the pocket." Whatever you call it, it's a state of mind that allows the body to do what it does best when it isn't being distracted from the critical, negative, judgmental influences of the conscious mind. Sometimes it can be contagious. Watch any audience member at a jazz virtuoso concert and you will see a group of mesmerized people, tapping their feet, picking at an imaginary guitar, or patting their thighs like they were a pair of congas, all with little or no conscious awareness of what they are doing.

The act of visualization, whether guided by another or self-directed, has been proven to be an effective means of enhancing personal performance in sports (Olsson, Jonsson & Nyberg, 2008; Silbernagel, Short, & Ross-Stewart, 2007), rehabilitation medicine (Muller, Butefisch, Seitz, & Homberg, 2007; Cramer, Orr, Cohen, & Lacourse, 2007), and personal behavior such as smoking cessation (Carmody et al., 2008; Elkins, Marcus, Bates, Hasau, Rajab, & Cook, 2006; Elkins & Rajab 2004) and weight management (Bolocofsky, Spinler, & Coulthard-Morris, 1985; Johnson, 1997).

In his Inner Game series (1973, 1981, 2000), Timothy Gallwey stresses three interrelated principles that he believes are essential for change, namely, awareness, choice, and trust. It is the third principle, trust, that enables an individual to move in a desired direction and that we are helping our clients' access through hypnotic interventions. Borrowing from Zen philosophy and humanistic psychology, Gallwey proposed that individual performance, whether on the tennis court, ski slopes, golf greens, or board room, involves an outer game and an inner game. Identifying Self 1 (conscious, critical, ego-invested) and Self 2 (subconscious resources of vast knowledge and abilities) as the primary components struggling to control the person, Gallwey built a theory and practice of performance enhancement around the notion that success can be potentiated by quieting Self 1 and *trusting* the silent intelligence of Self 2.

In our habit control work with our clients, our aim, like Gallwey's, is to enhance trust of the silent intelligence of the body. In his books, Gallwey helps his readers quiet Self 1 by trusting that Self 2 is very capable of accomplishing a goal without any guided instruction or critical correction of Self 1. Through hypnosis, we help our clients access the resources that are difficult to access consciously, because it is the unconscious mind that possesses the knowledge, abilities, and automatic physical responses that promote wanted change.

As we witness evidence suggesting the client is in trance, we invite the client to clearly and compellingly picture himself in his own future, *being* the person he wants to be. The more vividly he can perceive, feel, and experience himself in this new place and time, the greater the opportunity for enhancing subconscious resources that will allow the client to achieve the goals he seeks. Ultimately, by doing this, we are inviting the client to identify himself as a permanent nonsmoker, or as permanently fit and trim, and so on. At the same time, projecting into this future promotes inevitability as opposed to the doubt, criticism, and disbelief of the conscious mind that has (hitherto, successfully) challenged the client's ability to stop smoking or lose weight.

Eventually, we will have the client picture the path between how she is currently and the new self she seeks, as well as repeat the message associated with the gift that is her new self: "Look at *this Mary*, Mary the permanent nonsmoker. *This* 'Mary' is the gift of _____." And we again review all the reasons and the purpose of the goal, since purpose drives motivation.

And after we have the client successfully imagine moving down the path, we have him go through this process again, but this time encourage the client to get in touch with the feelings of moving down the path. During this experience, we can empower the client, foster a sense of strength, confidence, as he feels what it is like to be wearing the clothes he wants to wear, hearing the compliments others will say, feel himself moving around, seeing himself engaging in activities that include exercise, breathing easier, and, for the permanent nonsmoker, experiencing what it is like to have fresh-smelling clothes, homes, and cars, which are typically ashtray-scented.

When guiding our clients along this path, there are two important elements to keep in mind and include in trance work. The first involves content. It is important to consider what specific content the person requires for success. Having examined the information obtained from the assessments discussed in earlier chapters, including the Enneagram (chapter 3), we include the content that is relevant for our clients. It may be picturing—or feeling—themselves "eating healthy" or making good choices at the grocery store; it may be helping them access necessary resources that will enhance motivation for exercising; it may be identifying effective ways for managing stress; it may be finding new ways to deal with distracting triggers or cues for smoking. Additionally, as we provide the content to the client, we also want to minimize the threat of thinking that involves a "might have been" or "could have been" problem.

The second important element with guiding the client along her path involves themes through which the content is applied. For instance, we help the client see herself in the process of making certain decisions and doing so successfully. It is one thing to imagine doing something, but it is another to include thoughts and experiences that lead up to the behavior itself.

Along with imagined behaviors we want to include emotions and sensations in the hypnotherapy work. We want the client to feel all of the benefits of being this permanently slim and fit person, this permanent nonsmoker. We not only want the person to be more active or have more energy, we want the emotions that go along with that experience as well. We can invite the person in trance to imagine how it feels to be more energetic or more vibrant, have more vitality, and be motivated to keep their eyes on the prize he seeks.

Many clients place contingencies on life decisions and in some ways these contingencies have limited their capacity to achieve their goals. For some, this is initiating an exercise regimen, or starting a new diet, or making this the last cigarette. When life presents an unexpected stressor, or someone offers them a cigarette, or the cheesecake at a favorite restaurant is irresistible, the best laid intentions crumble like a house of cards in a wind storm.

In an effort to minimize the unexpected detractors, we help our clients develop a "no matter what" philosophy that reinforces their resolve to become a permanent nonsmoker and/or permanently fit and trim individual. We want to avoid what Brian refers to as greenhouse hypnosis or therapy. In a greenhouse, plants thrive with drip irrigation, filtered lighting, misting, etc. But once the plant is purchased and taken home, it must survive despite the real-world threats of cool drafts, forgotten watering, or pets that nip at leaves. Our clients' success should not be "as long as" or "until" or "when" or "if this or that." Such perspectives undermine the permanence that we stress with our clients and place limits on the work that is done. Instead, we want to promote success *no matter what*. So in the course of our hypnosis work we will say things like, "You can see yourself down this path, in your future, the permanently slim and fit Judy, no matter what. No matter where you are, no matter what you're doing, no matter who you are with, you can see and feel the permanently slim and fit you."

CONCLUSION

In this chapter we initially offered suggestions for ways to introduce hypnosis to your client, especially for circumstances in which a client may be resistant, reluctant, or intimidated by their understanding of hypnosis. We also introduced you to a number of hypnotic procedures or strategies that enhance the efficacy of trance for your client, including presupposition, use of contextual cues, descriptive matching, splitting, linking, and the more advanced technique of interspersal. Using a GPS metaphor, we offered some pragmatic suggestions for organizing and implementing a hypnosis session. Finally, borrowing Bill O'Hanlon's "Class of Problems/Class of Solutions" Model, we identified specific hypnotic interventions based on a client's presenting concern. By using this model you will be able to conceptualize appropriate interventions that can be tailored to help your clients manage unwanted behavior.

Things to Do

1. Introduce hypnosis to a friend, colleague, or family member who has little or no understanding of hypnosis.
2. Use splitting, interspersal, linking, and presupposition during your practice sessions.
3. Seek a "friendly" volunteer who is willing and perhaps eager to go into trance with your guidance. Pay particular attention to the sound and rhythm of your voice as

you match your volunteer's breathing. Hypnosis is like learning to play an instrument: with practice you will establish your own rhythm and become more comfortable and confident.

10 Mindfulness: Minding Your Habits

People will do anything, no matter how absurd, to avoid facing their own soul.

—Carl Jung

So much of our habit behavior is automatic and unthinking. Smokers often say, "I didn't even know I was smoking" or "I put one out and lit up another one without realizing it." The chronic, or even not-so-chronic overeater will profess, "I can't believe I ate all that."

Consider for a moment the number of times you engage in mindless behavior. Perhaps while driving you've missed a turn or ended up in the wrong place knowing your intended destination was elsewhere. We've all been guilty of walking into a room and suddenly becoming amnestic as to the reason for our visit to the room. It's as if we were unknowingly placed in some kind of trance that promoted a sense of disorientation as we entered the room and announced to everyone present that we haven't a clue what we are doing there. When was the last time you tied your shoes? Did you actually think of every fine movement that was essential for correctly tying your shoe? We sure hope not!

In many ways, human behavior involves this kind of absent-minded thinking. For this reason, nearly every program for psychological, spiritual, or habit-control treatment incorporates some element of mindfulness. Of course, mindfulness to every little thing we do throughout the day can likely lead to momentary insanity and would be ill advised. Nonetheless, it is important to cultivate conscientious awareness and conscious choice. In a way, it is like informed decision making that typically precedes any proposed medical intervention, like taking a certain kind of medication or undergoing some surgical intervention.

Mindfulness is the practice of present-moment awareness and experiencing without judgment. When engaging in mindfulness, we can expect to experience a number of potential difficulties as well as wonderful insights. With growing awareness in each moment, in situations of our lives, we become aware of the unpleasant and painful as well as the pleasant. It is equally plausible that we can acquire a greater appreciation of the "neutral" in our lives, and with greater recognition of these moments gain a sense of some unpleasant or pleasant aspect previously unnoticed. Either way, mindfulness involves a waking-up to the reality of our lives. Yet, with all of the inherent distractions in life (both within our minds and from external stimuli), it can be challenging to remain mindful for an extended period of time. For this reason, we teach and encourage our clients to practice daily meditation. These meditative experiences are not to replace hypnosis; the two, though seemingly comparable, are in actuality, very different. The former involves self-directed, effortful mindfulness, while the latter consists of passive, unconscious processing with the guided assistance of another.

Through mindfulness practice, such as meditation or yoga, we encourage our clients to become aware of any internalized pain or discomfort while noticing their reaction to this experience. Far too frequently, people react to this pain with a spirit of criticism, meanness, or sense of personal failure. This, in turn, leads to destructive patterns of behavior that only exacerbates the misery already felt. Teaching our clients to embrace this pain with kindness and compassion instead of harsh judgment or criticism helps them take a different attitude toward their emotional pain and suffering. By replacing unhealthy habits involving self-destructive behaviors, we help our clients develop habits of kindness, compassion, and composure in the face of crisis or difficult life experiences.

In our experience, mindful meditation helps our clients develop an acceptance of what is while offering hope for what can be. One poignant example of this is the Serenity Prayer, which asks for the serenity to accept the things we cannot change, courage to change the things we can, and most importantly, the wisdom to know the difference.

The opposite of conscious choice is *mindlessness*. It is the "automatic pilot" that guides our reactions to stress until we experience the physical, emotional, or psychological consequences of our mindlessness. A plethora of destructive reactions, including muscle tension, panic, depression, obsessive ruminations, self-criticism, smoking, and overeating can manifest themselves. An important antidote to this "tuning out" is to practice mindfulness.

Practicing mindfulness requires effort and intention. To start the process, we introduce our clients to mindfulness by starting our sessions with two minutes of silence and focused attention to our breathing. We may then have them focus on their breathing during the session, making them mindful of how their bodies are responding, feeling, and behaving. Mindfulness can be practiced at any time. Whether we are sitting at a red light, eating a meal, walking the dog, people watching, or washing the dishes, we can practice mindfulness by gently paying attention to our breath, to the sounds and sights around us, or just to our thoughts.

Conscious choice is the natural byproduct of mindfulness that allows us to consider the decisions we are about to make. When used appropriately and effectively, it gives us a moment to pause and consider the implications of our behaviors. For instance, you may be watching a television program one evening and consider eating some chocolate mint chip ice cream. Some of you may be thinking that sounds like a great idea now as you read this last sentence. Either way, if you were to pause a moment, consider the choice you are about to make and all of the implications of that decision, you would be engaging in more conscious choice and thereby making a more informed decision about making that choice. You could, for instance, consider first and foremost whether you actually are hungry. Then you could consider the calories, fat grams, or carbohydrates that would be consumed, as well as the resulting glycemic index. Perhaps you may even think about the last time you exercised and whether or not consuming ice cream would be defeating the purpose of exercising that day, the day before, or even tomorrow.

FOUR IMPORTANT QUESTIONS TO DETERMINE WHAT AND HOW MUCH TO EAT

It never ceases to amaze us how readily people can calibrate hunger. They may state that they are "getting a little hungry" or "getting hungrier" or are "starved" or "famished." Based on these "feelings," people may then consume food to the extent that it leads to overeating. Interestingly, this calibration doesn't seem to go in the opposite direction. Rarely will you hear someone say, "I'm getting a little full" or "I'm feeling fuller now." Rather, we just continue to eat until at some point we proclaim that we ate too much and are "stuffed."

We can liken this lack of calibration to an automobile without gauges or even "idiot" lights that alert us to the slightest automotive concern. Without these sensors, we might never find out that our car was about to overheat until the hood pops and steam rolls off the engine. Or, perhaps more to the point, imagine not having an automatic shut-off mechanism at the gasoline pump. How often would we insert the spout into the gas tank, squeeze the handle, and head inside to pay for our purchase only to return moments later to find gasoline spewing like a geyser and realize that "our tank runneth over"?

Though bizarre indeed when considering an overflowing gas tank, that is the very thing that most of us do when eating. With this in mind, we offer five important questions to determine what and how much to eat. Questions that are designed to help us enhance awareness and conscious choice, which, again, is critical for successful habit control.

Question #1: Am I Hungry?

Many people just assume that, if they are about to eat something, they must be hungry. But more often than we may think, we eat for reasons other than to satiate feelings of hunger. This very question cultivates awareness about our present state of being. It begs the question: "What is going on?" And sometimes we may conclude that we are hungry, but often we may be thirsty instead and should chose a beverage, preferably a low-calorie drink, instead of a bag of potato chips or a bowl of ice cream.

Question #2: If I Am Not Hungry, Why Do I Want to Eat?

If a person concludes that he is not hungry, he should be encouraged to consider alternatives to whatever it was that led him to the refrigerator or food pantry. There may be underlying emotions that need tending to. Perhaps the person is stressed and looking for some food to settle the nerves. Maybe he is lonely or bored and needs to feel full in some way that makes him feel something other than loneliness and/or boredom.

If bored, we encourage our clients to find something to do. Usually we prepare our clients for this by having them consider things they can do once they feel bored. They should have the options of activities readily available to them, rather than have to seek something out once they get to a place of boredom. If this is not successful, we encourage them to simply maintain that boredom, as eating is the third and last resort to alleviating their boredom.

We are "undoing" the automatic connection that exists between boredom (or some other feeling) and eating. This is not to say that we oppose eating just for the enjoyment of eating. Consumption of food can and should be an enjoyed experience. However, like anything in life, too much of a good thing can become destructive, so we encourage moderation. Unfortunately, too many people with weight concerns have an automatic response of eating food for reasons other than hunger.

Question #3: How Will Eating This Food Make Me Feel Emotionally and Physically Immediately After Eating It, 2 Minutes From Now, 10 Minutes From Now, and 30 Minutes From Now?

Whether consciously intended or not, we are always preparing our future. Everything we do ultimately leads to our future. Whether we go for a walk, take a nap, sit and read a book, consume a meal, or smoke a cigarette, all behavior has relevance for our future. Recall how, in chapter 6, we discussed the importance of establishing a timeline and utilized it as a means of movement down the path? If we examine our timeline for the last 3 months concerning food and exercise, there is only one conclusion: It is obvious that we are the way we are now. Because of the decisions we have made, our bodies couldn't possibly be any other way.

If we go beyond that time to 6 months hence, we will likely be saying the very same thing: "Of course, I gained another 10 pounds. I've been vegetating on the couch, didn't exercise, and ate fried chicken, greasy burgers, and French fries. Or perhaps we will be able to say, to the contrary, "Of course my body's in great shape. I ate healthfully, exercised several days per week, and lost weight."

Because we are always preparing our future, why not take this opportunity to have our conscious say what future we want and do all that we can to make sure that happens? Besides, how often do you find yourself saying, "Oh, I shouldn't have eaten all that"? Asking the question "How will eating this food make me feel emotionally and physically over the course of the next several minutes?" affords ourselves the opportunity to try this out in our heads, perhaps more consciously, and enhances the possibility of making a better choice.

Question #4: Will Eating This Food in This Amount Move Me Closer to or Further Away From Becoming the Permanently Slim and Fit Person I Want to Be?

We have spent a considerable amount of time discussing this permanently slim and fit person and reviewed and demonstrated how we use hypnosis to move people down the path. This question offers the opportunity to calibrate hunger and make conscious choices on this path. By being aware and making good choices, we can take responsibility and accountability for our bodies.

MINIMALLY SATISFYING AMOUNT

The Minimally Satisfying Amount, or MSA, is the estimated amount of food or drink that would be considered minimally satisfying. For instance, if you had a 12-ounce can of 7-Up each day with lunch, and one day you were given a 10-ounce can instead, you would probably be okay with this smaller portion. But if, on the contrary, one day you were given a 2-ounce portion instead, you likely would not find that acceptable. This just might not be enough to quench your thirst or enjoy with your meal. At some point, you will reach and be able to identify the minimally satisfying amount.

By no means do we want to encourage obsessive calculations or estimations of MSA, as it wouldn't be feasible to instruct clients to consume one forkful of food at a time until they reach their MSA. We do, however, want to foster a greater sense of awareness and mindfulness of what one's MSA might be.

Surely, there is some point below which nutritional deprivation sets in and an individual remains uncomfortably hungry. But helping a person remain aware of a sense of satiation as they reach or come close to reaching the MSA facilitates a more conscious choice between not eating any more versus consuming more food. Once an individual has reached this minimally satisfying amount, she can consider giving all of the additional calories away as a gift to herself in the form of weight loss.

VOLUMETRICS: FEELING FULLER FASTER

We have already reviewed ways to evaluate healthy foods, times of day to eat, and even how to eat. Now we want to introduce you to a strategy for maximizing calories in terms of satisfaction and fullness. Volumetrics (simply stated, the study of fullness) was introduced by Dr. Barbara Rolls of Pennsylvania State University.

Dr. Rolls is a veteran nutrition researcher who has focused her research on the study of hunger and obesity. It is a fairly well established fact that the reason most people abandon diets only to return to unhealthy dietary habits is the lingering sense of hunger. In her book *The Volumetrics Eating Plan: Techniques and Recipes for Feeling Full on Fewer Calories* (2005), Dr. Rolls explains the key to feeling full: energy density of foods. Energy density is simply the concentration of calories in a given weight or serving size of food. The energy density of a particular food can be calculated by dividing the number of calories by the number of grams (cal/g). For instance, if a 28-g serving of a reduced-fat cheese stick is worth 60 calories, its energy density would be 2.1 (60/28 = 2.1). By the same token, a one-cup or 245-g serving of low-fat yogurt is worth 154 calories, with a resultant energy density of 0.61. The *lower* the number, the *better* the food, and the more of it you can consume without gaining weight. Obviously in the above two examples, a cup of low-fat yogurt is relatively better than a 28-g serving of a reduced-fat cheese stick.

Essentially, a food that is high in energy density has a large number of calories in a small amount of food, whereas a food with low energy density has fewer calories for the same weight of food. Consequently, according to Dr. Rolls' research, if we choose foods that offer fewer calories for the *same amount of food*, we will be able to manage our weight more effectively without going hungry.

To make matters more practical, consider this question: Will you feel fuller on two cups of grapes or one quarter-cup of raisins? One is simply a dried version of the other and both are worth the same number of calories (about 100 calories), but you could consume far more grapes because of their higher water content. Water has weight but no calories; consequently, the higher the moisture content of a given food, the lower its energy density, and the more of it you can consume allowing you to feel fuller without exponentially increasing caloric intake.

More recently, Dr. Rolls, along with her colleague J. E. Flood-Obbagy (2009), evaluated how apples in different forms consumed prior to a meal (e.g., apple, applesauce, and apple juice with and without added fiber) influence satiety and energy intake at meals. The preloads were all matched according to weight, energy content, energy density, and ingestion rate. Results of their study indicated that fullness ratings differed significantly among the preloads (apple > applesauce > both juices > control group), thereby supporting earlier research findings concerning volumetrics.

It should be noted that water or liquid alone does not seem to have the same lasting effect as when water is within the food. Consequently, what we are aiming for is food with a certain density, a certain weight with fewer calories.

Broccoli, for example, has low energy density and one could never gain weight eating copious amounts of broccoli (not that we would recommend it). Because of the fiber, water content, and weight, there would be relatively quick satisfaction, especially for the caloric intake. For this reason, having broccoli and other vegetables with a low-fat dip is recommended for enhancing satiety and reducing the likelihood of overeating the main course.

Potato chips, on the other hand, are very light in weight but high in calories. Consequently, as a shrewd marketing slogan puts it, "you can't eat just one" to be satiated. Manufacturers of potato chips are well aware of this and use it to their advantage when marketing their product. Consider the number of people watching a football game while mindlessly stuffing their mouths with handfuls of potato chips until they reach the bottom of an empty bag. So, in this case, it isn't satisfaction or fullness that stops the feeding frenzy, it's the lack of food available. And in the end, a tremendous amount of calories has been ingested and the person may still feel hungry.

BEING MINDFUL OF DEPRIVATION

As discussed previously, mindfulness involves being aware of all that is happening in the present moment, without implied judgment. This present-moment awareness can involve pleasant and unpleasant thoughts and sensations. We may agree in principle that the notion of deprivation is uncomfortable and unwanted, as its very definition according to *Webster's New World Dictionary* (2001) is "to keep from having, using, or enjoying." It therefore goes without saying that most people focus on what they are giving up and not what they are receiving when they are being deprived. The last thing they are considering is the possible benefit of giving something up.

Recall our scenario of the decision between eating a Snickers bar versus no Snickers bar or smoking a cigarette versus no cigarette at all. As we observed, the decision is not between a Snickers bar and no Snickers bar or a cigarette and no cigarette, it is between the Snickers bar/cigarette and the permanently slim and fit person one wants to be, with all the attributes, benefits, and blessings of a healthier, permanently nonsmoking person. Employing such a reframing and mindful reflecting about one's body, the Snickers bar or cigarette is suddenly not much of a treat at all.

The NIC Fit

When it comes to the uncomfortable physical sensation of nicotine withdrawal, we again emphasize mindfulness of the experience. In addition to using hypnosis and energy psychology, which we will expand upon in the next chapter, maintaining a level of mindfulness and cognitive reframing can facilitate a more comfortable response to nicotine withdrawal, especially if nicotine replacement is not being used.

Although some clients may not require this information, at times, it is challenging to ascertain which clients would benefit from it and which clients may take the information as a negative suggestion or presupposition that only promotes the very behavior they are trying to minimize or avoid. Consequently, when discussing nicotine withdrawal, we couch it in rather conservative and generalized terms.

We tell them the following: "Realize that not all smokers experiences nicotine withdrawal when they quit smoking, and you might not either. But for those people who have some problems with this" [and here we actually point and turn to the side of the person as if we were talking about someone else], "I would tell them, 'If you had some sense of irritability or some strange sensation like feeling as if your skin were crawling, you know what that means? It's your body's way of telling you that the toxins are coming out.' So, you can just say, 'Ah, the toxins are leaving my body. Good riddance.' "

It can also be helpful to have our clients consider their lifeline and the path they are creating in front of them by making changes now. Despite the potential discomfort, by having them consider how much time they have left to live and the relatively little time they will experience discomfort, we can help them focus on their healthier future.

So we tell them, "Let's consider how much time, within reasonable expectations, you have left to live if you were to stop smoking. As a 35-year-old man, you could reasonably live another 40 years. So, if we create a life path in front of us" [and here we point to a place in front of the person], "in which each year is a foot and each month is an inch, we can create a 40-foot life path right here. And because you may have struggled with or had to deal with some discomfort for the first quarter of an inch of this new time line, and the next 44 feet and 13/16 of an inch are going to offer you a greater quality of health, enhanced energy, better sense of self, and personal mastery, just consider what an incredible return you'll have on your investment."

We also remind our clients of the times they caught a cold and felt very uncomfortable. None of us when suffering from the symptoms of a head cold become so despondent that we are at risk for developing a major depressive disorder because of it. Though it is a big nuisance to have a cold and it is a big deal when we are in the middle of an illness, we know that when we sneeze and wheeze and our head aches and our throat is scratchy it will all resolve in due time; usually a matter of days to a week. The symptoms will resolve and we will soon feel better and forget that we were even sick.

Some of our clients have such extensive histories of cigarette smoking that they may have a longer relationship with cigarettes than with any person in their life. In these cases, they may consider cigarettes as their "best friend."

In these cases we tell our clients, "If you had someone in your life who you thought was a good friend for many years, but you find out that this person has been vandalizing your home and embezzling your money, what would you do with this so-called friend? Would you decide it was time for him to be out of your life? Regardless of how much fun and companionship he had given you in the past, wouldn't you want him to leave?

Wouldn't you walk the person to the door and show him the way out? And if this vandal, this embezzler starts knocking on your door, you are not going to give him the keys to your house, are you? Would you hand over your checkbook so he'd stop knocking on your door? Of course not. You're going to get rid of the person for good. So you can do the same with your old pal, Marlboro/Winston/Kool."

"Clean The Plate"

Most of our weight-control clients present with persistent issues that involve a compulsion to clean their plates and eat everything in front of them. There are many reasons for this behavior that may date to early childhood food deprivation, early indoctrination regarding the need to fight for food, childhood experiences in which the person learned to comfort herself with food, or any of several other possibilities. Whatever the reason, it clearly impedes portion control and prohibits the mindfulness that leads to conscious choice.

To help people become more mindful of their eating behaviors, we encourage them to imagine that, while they are eating, someone else approaches them and asks them if they are planning to eat what is left on their plate, as if it were available for anyone to consume. If they respond to that inquiry by saying "No, go right ahead, help yourself," that should be a cue that they do not *have to* finish what is on their plate.

We also introduce them to a rather silly, but effective way to minimize compulsive and unnecessary consumption of food. We introduce them to the "Brown Bag Intervention." We set things up by telling them that we have a foolproof way to prevent compulsive eating, but before we share this secret with them we obtain their agreement to follow through with the intervention. We tell them how much we appreciate our society's concerns about solid waste removal and that they will now be sacrificing themselves and using their own bodies as a waste receptacle rather than throwing unconsumed food down the drain.

We then introduce them to the Brown Bag Intervention, which involves the use of a large plastic garbage bag. We instruct them to cut four big holes in the bag for their arms and legs and have them wear this bag whenever they are going to eat food after reaching the minimally satisfying amount. Essentially, if they were to eat more food simply because it is there on their plate or available to eat despite feeling satiated, they must engage in congruent behavior and wear the garbage bag. We take it a step further and invite them to purchase different-colored bags for different occasions, such as holidays or when visiting friends or relatives.

It has been our experience that this can be very powerful despite the fact that they never wear the bag. Just having this image in mind when they eat can deter them from overeating. Also, because they have "promised" us that they will do this, they might not put the bag on, but will most likely follow through on the agreement and not overeat. This intervention also gives them another image in their mind that can help facilitate awareness and choice.

By remaining mindful of the choices before us and learning alternative ways to reframe and reconsider uncomfortable withdrawal symptoms, we can help our clients enhance the likelihood that they will become permanent nonsmokers and permanently physically fit individuals.

As you will see in the next chapter, on energy psychology or, more specifically, Emotional Freedom Techniques, we can help our clients clear any unwanted physical or emotional symptoms.

CONCLUSION

In this chapter we introduced the concept of mindfulness. The practice of present-moment awareness and experiencing without judgment that leads to conscious choice can enhance a client's sense of control over their unwanted behavior and build confidence that they can overcome any possible uncomfortable physical or emotional sensations. We offered four simple questions for our clients with weight-management concerns that promote conscious choice and move them further down the path toward achieving their desired goal: "Am I hungry?" "If not, why do I want to eat?" "How will this food make me feel?" and "Will eating this food bring me closer or further away from the trim and fit body I desire?"

We also introduced the concept of a Minimally Satisfying Amount of food and an understanding of food volumetrics for enhancing satiety while keeping caloric consumption under control. For many of our weight management clients, understanding volumetrics allows them to make better informed decisions regarding their daily dietary consumption.

Finally, we discussed and reviewed some mindful interventions that help manage a sense of deprivation and physical discomfort associated with smoking cessation in addition to offering guidelines for assisting clients with compulsions to overeat.

Things to Do

1. Spend 5 to 10 minutes each day for 1 week engaging in mindfulness meditation and note how well you are able to remain present-focused, how much time you spend being critical and judgmental, and how much time you are able to be accepting of what is. Encourage at least one client to do the same for one week.

2. Introduce at least one client to the four questions about what and how much to eat and have them report back to you how successful this was for curbing their dietary consumption, particularly at times when they determined that they were seeking food but were not hungry.

3. Review the concept of volumetrics with at least one client. Have your client evaluate the volumetrics of the food they consume and encourage them to consider other food sources with lower energy density.

4. Identify a client who desires to become a permanent nonsmoker and review the timeline discussed above to help them become more mindful of their capacity to manage uncomfortable feelings associated with nicotine withdrawal.

11 Energy Psychology and Emotional Freedom Techniques

Energy and persistence alter all things.

—Benjamin Franklin

ENERGY PSYCHOLOGY

Expanding on conventional therapeutic interventions, Energy Psychology uses techniques from acupressure, yoga, qi gong, and energy medicine that teach people simple steps for initiating change in their lives. Energy Psychology works by stimulating energy points on the surface of the skin, which, when paired with specific psychological principles, can alter the brain's electrochemistry, which in turn allows a person to change unwanted habits and behaviors (see Furman & Gallo, 2000; Gallo, 2005).

Although still controversial within the mental health field, evidence supporting the pragmatic benefits of Energy Psychology has increased over the past few years (see Feinstein & Eden, 2008; Garakani, Mathew, & Charney, 2006; Meyers, 2007; Rowe, 2005). Despite these advances, much research is still needed to provide a greater understanding of the underlying mechanisms of Energy Psychology. As a consequence, some of the techniques utilized to remove obstacles that challenge permanent habit control have limited "face validity" and will require a level of "buy-in" for some of your clients. Many mental health professionals and organizations, including the American Psychological Association, have yet to fully approve and endorse continuing education units for seminars on Emotional Freedom Techniques (EFT) or Energy Psychology. Though the jury is still out on Energy Psychology, we have included it as part of this text because we have been overwhelmingly impressed with the benefits of Energy Psychology, and EFT in particular, for habit control.

Energy Psychology involves three interrelated systems, including energy pathways (meridians), energy centers (chakras), and the human biofield (aura). For the purposes of this text, we will predominantly focus on energy meridians and acupoints (locations on the body that are the focus of acupuncture and acupressure) associated with those meridians.

Meridians are essentially energy channels that can be likened to the wiring of a house or the veins and arteries of the body through which blood flows, except that meridians lack any discrete physical structure and cannot be dissected or found surgically. These pressure-point areas can be stimulated to generate healing or, as David has learned in his Kempo Karate class, to employ significant pain and discomfort in ways that promote self-defense (Torite Jutsu).

Meridians are part of the body's subtle energy anatomy, yet lack physical form. It is believed that all living mammals have energy meridians. Despite their intangible form, we know they exist because they can be felt. Sedating or stimulating certain meridians promotes a noticeable change in energy levels, mood, overall health, thinking, and emotional stability.

There are 14 meridians that have been identified by traditional Chinese medicine. Stressful events in our lives and negative or pessimistic thinking can affect the energy system throughout our body and result in anxiety, depression, fear, and anger. It is believed that the energy of these emotions can become lodged in our body's physical and energy systems, thereby creating blockages within the meridians. Through Energy Psychology principles, we apply pressure to or gently tap the meridian points while verbalizing positive affirmations to release these destructive emotions from the physical body.

Manual muscle testing, or applied kinesiology, is a noninvasive way of gathering information from the body about what is happening internally. Some refer to muscle testing as "energy testing," since the kind of feedback received during the testing has nothing to do with the strength of muscles and everything to do with the energy of the body. We, however, prefer the term muscle testing and will use that term throughout this chapter.

Muscle testing has also been used to identify allergies, physical weaknesses, and nutritional deficiencies and to assess what kinds of supplements or other treatments may be beneficial for the body (Lawson & Calderon, 1997; Schmitt & Leisman, 1998; Vinci, Serrao, Pierelli, Sandrini, & Santilli, 2006), though there are ample method skeptics who question the validity of such procedures for the assessment of medical conditions (Beyer & Teuber, 2005; Hall, Lewith, Brien, & Little, 2008; Wurthrich, 2005). Interestingly, and as an aside, one evening during a karate class, David noticed an area of sensitivity near the underside of his left wrist. Though others in the class did not appear to have the same level of sensitivity, David asked his fifth-degree black belt instructor about his apparent hypersensitivity. Turns out that this particular meridian connects with the lungs, and David indeed has exercise- and allergy-induced asthma.

The typical form of muscle testing requires one person to act as the evaluator, and one as the client. The client extends an arm (or leg, depending on the muscle being tested) in the proper position and attempts to hold it firmly in place without "locking" the muscle or forcing their arm upward, while the tester applies gentle pressure to move the limb in a prescribed range of motion. The general guideline is to use two fingers and about two pounds of pressure for testing.

If a muscle holds firm, the related organ or system is strong and healthy. If the client is unable to hold firm and their arm moves under gentle pressure, the muscle's related organ or system requires strengthening via energy work.

Because every person will demonstrate a slightly different and perhaps unique way of showing strong and weak responses, it is important to "calibrate" before testing. The most common muscle used for testing is the anterior deltoid (see Figure 11.1), whereby the client extends an arm to the side or straight out in front of the body, parallel to the floor. The tester then asks a question that will yield a yes-or-no response and the person is instructed to be honest at times and dishonest at other times. There should be a noticeable difference between honest and dishonest answers. For example, we could ask a man, "Are you a woman?" and when replying "Yes" to the question his arm would likely readily give way to the pressure applied. Answering "No" to the question should produce a much stronger reaction and an arm that is not easily moved. Alternatively, the tester could ask the person nonsense questions like "Is grass purple?" or "Can dogs fly?" or "Does five plus five equal nine?" and note the difference in muscle testing between both "yes" and "no" responses.

At times, we encounter clients whose muscle response is the exact opposite of what we expect. For instance, David was working with Nancy, a 38-year-old overweight woman, who for years had tried to lose weight. No matter what diet, exercise, or weight loss plan she followed, Nancy was unable to keep the weight off. Typically, whenever starting a new plan, she would lose about 20 pounds, only to see it return within a matter of months. She tried Curves, Weight Watchers, the South Beach diet, and, most recently before consulting with David, The Atkins Diet. During the initial consultation with David, Nancy reported a desire to lose 100 pounds in 1 year. She informed him that if this "last ditch effort" failed, she was going to consider gastric bypass surgery.

During muscle testing with Nancy, as expected, David was able to ascertain a positive response to the calibration questions (e.g., Are you a woman? Is your name Nancy? Is grass purple? Can dogs fly?). To his utter shock and surprise, when responding, "Yes" to the question, "Do you want to lose weight?" Nancy's arm failed to resist the applied pressure, suggesting there was a significant discrepancy between her verbal response to the question and her physical reaction. To further assess the situation, David had Nancy say aloud, "I want to lose weight" while applying gentle pressure to her arm. The test indicated that her statement was untrue. He then had her say, "I want to gain weight" and, despite the look on her face which suggested otherwise, her arm resisted the applied pressure. This, of course, was quite upsetting to Nancy, who felt she was doomed to failure no matter what she tried to do to lose weight.

Unfortunately, there are times when a client's verbalized desire to change and the body's response to muscle testing are incongruous, as in Nancy's case. Dr. Roger Callahan (1990), sometimes called the founding father of EFT, called this response *psychological reversal*.

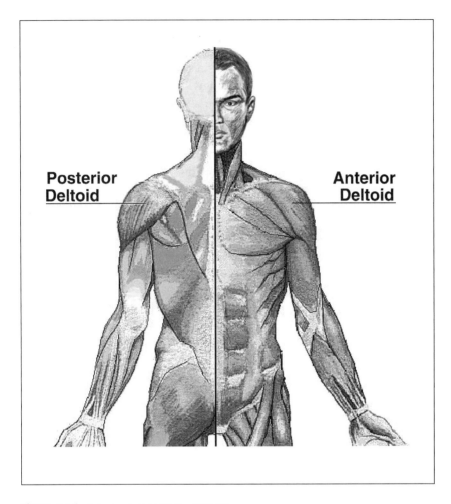

Figure 11.1 Anterior and posterior deltoids.

The principle cause of psychological reversal (PR) is negative thinking. Even the best of optimistic thinkers have moments of subconscious negative thinking that involves self-defeating thought patterns and interferes with optimal functioning. Consider the future Hall of Fame baseball player who struggles in a batting slump that at the time seems endless. Generally speaking, the more pervasive the negative thinking, the more prone an individual is to become psychologically reversed.

For some it seems a lifelong struggle as they become victims to the world and everything in it. For them "nothing works," or so they believe.

According to Callahan, PR is not a character defect, but an indication that one suffers from a chronic reversal of the electrical polarities in one's body. This person's energy systems literally work against him as if his batteries were in backwards. For most people, PR is present in select areas of their lives, such as consciously desiring to lose weight, stop smoking, or change other unwanted habits. For the smoker who consciously reports a strong desire to quit smoking, he may give up the habit for a while only to sabotage his own efforts and start smoking again because he is PR.

Psychological reversal is correctable, according to Callahan and other proponents of EFT. The process of reversing PR allows the body's natural healing processes to work more fluidly by adjusting the energy flow through the entire body. It is important to note that when PR is present, the standard "tapping" principles of EFT will not work properly; consequently, as with Nancy, it was essential to adjust the PR before implementing any interventions that would help her in her quest to lose weight.

In the standard procedures for EFT, an "automatic correction" is included. Consequently, one does not necessarily need to test for PR, though, at times, it is helpful to verify that this is a possible impediment to successful habit control. The correction involves a neutralizing verbalized affirmation of the problem confronted by the individual, which will be addressed again below as we review the procedures for EFT.

EFT involves several steps for unblocking the energy that is interfering with desired progress. Gary Craig, who authored an EFT manual that is available for free download at www.emofree.com, offers what he refers to as "The Basic Recipe" for EFT and will be briefly summarized here. Like Craig, we encourage you to consider additional training experiences through the demonstration videos that are available at the above-mentioned Web site. We are, however, compelled to report that although Craig and several of his colleagues, despite their cautionary statements, profess EFT as a treatment for nearly every kind of physical and/or emotional ailment, we have found it to be selectively beneficial for treating individuals desiring to quit smoking or become permanently fit and trim. Consequently, our discussion and application of EFT for habit control in this text is not necessarily indicative of an endorsement of these procedures for treating all other psychological or physical illnesses as espoused by Craig through his Web site or instructional materials.

EFT Procedures

The primary procedures of EFT consist of four steps, as follows:

1. The Setup
2. The Sequence
3. The Nine Gamut Procedure
4. The Sequence Again

1. The Setup

1. Repeat an affirmation three times while you....
2. Rub the "Sore Spot" or, alternatively, tap the "Karate Chop" point (see Figures 11.2 and 11.3).

The affirmation consists of saying aloud "Even though I have this (craving for a cigarette/difficulty losing weight), I deeply and completely accept myself." Your client can use whatever words they deem fit for addressing the possible PR that is potentially impeding progress. These affirmations follow a general format that acknowledges the problem and creates self-acceptance despite the existence of the problem.

We have found that the affirmation is more effective when stated out loud with feeling and emphasis; however, we understand there are times when an individual may not be in the most ideal circumstances to do so. Stating it silently to oneself is acceptable, though not preferable.

The Setup involves either the simultaneous rubbing of the "Sore Spot" or tapping on the "Karate Chop" point while repeating the affirmation three times with emphasis. There are two Sore Spots, and either is fine to use for this step in the sequence. They are located in the upper left and right portions of the chest. To find them, place the index and middle fingers of both hands at the base of the throat, about where the knot of a necktie would rest. You will find a "U" shaped notch at the top of your sternum or breastbone. From the top of that notch go down about 3 inches toward your navel and over 3 inches to your left and right. You should now be in the upper left and right

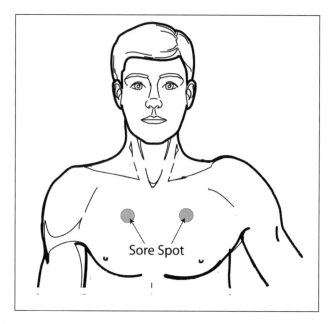

Figure 11.2 Sore spots.

portion of your chest. If you press vigorously in that area (within a 2-inch radius) you will feel two areas that may appear sensitive or "sore." These are the sore spots (see Figure 11.2).

This spot is sore when you rub it vigorously because lymphatic congestion occurs here. When you rub and put pressure on the area, you are essentially dispersing congestion. After a few episodes of rubbing the congestion is dispersed and you will notice that the soreness goes away. Henceforth, you can rub the sore spot areas without any subsequent discomfort, provided of course, you don't go several weeks to months without clearing the congestion. We tell our clients that the pain in this area is typically indicative of some level of energy blocking that needs clearing and in some ways serves as a sort of "litmus test" for any potential disruption to energy flow.

A Sore Spot on either or both sides can be rubbed; however, if your client has greater pain sensitivity on one side or has had some surgical or medical procedure that creates discomfort or prohibits rubbing that area, using the "healthier" side is advised.

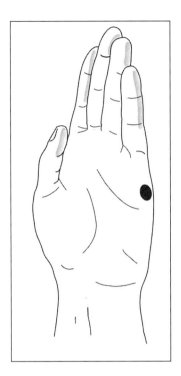

Figure 11.3 Karate chop point (note the marking).

The Karate Chop (KC) point (see Figure 11.3) is located at the center of the fleshy part of the outside of either hand between the top of the wrist and the base of the pinky. Essentially, it is the part of the hand that is uses for delivering a karate chop. Rather than rub this area as you would the Sore Spot, you vigorously tap it with the fingertips of the index and middle fingers of the opposite hand. One could also karate chop the side of the index finger of the opposite hand as it too is held in a karate chop position (see Figure 11.4).

You could use the Karate Chop point of either hand, though most people find it more comfortable to "tap" their nondominant hand with their dominant hand index and middle fingers. We prefer using the Karate Chop method depicted in Figure 11.4 by chopping the nondominant hand (left) with the dominant hand (right).

With regard to which method is more effective for undoing PR, Gary Craig reports that "After years of experiencing with both methods,

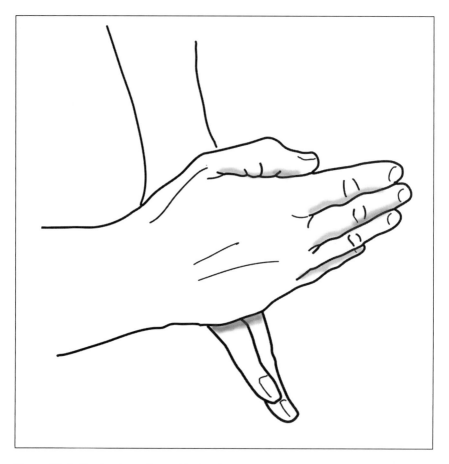

Figure 11.4 Karate chop of opposite hand.

it has been determined that rubbing the Sore Spot is a bit more effective than tapping the Karate Chop point. It doesn't have a commanding lead by any means, but it *is* preferred (p. 23, EFT manual available for free download at www.emofree.com). We would agree with this opinion, as it has been our own experience that the Sore Spot is the preferred method for addressing PR. The Sore Spot, unlike the KC, offers an assessment of blocked energy clearing efficacy through any experienced physical discomfort or lack thereof when rubbing this area.

After you or your client repeat the affirmation three times while either rubbing the Sore Spot or tapping/chopping the KC, then the next step, referred to as The Sequence, can be initiated.

2. The Sequence

The Sequence is a rather simple concept and easy to learn and commit to memory. It involves tapping the end points of energy meridians in the body and is the primary method by which the energy system is balanced out. Before identifying the specific meridian points, we will first review the process of tapping.

Tips for Tapping: You can tap with either or even both hands simultaneously, though we have found it to be more convenient to tap with your dominant hand. Although Gary Craig recommends tapping with only the index and middle fingers, it really is a matter of personal preference, as we have found using the first three fingers to be more effective for ensuring that the meridian point is appropriately stimulated. Tapping should be done with solid pressure, though never so hard as to hurt or bruise yourself. We recommend tapping about seven (7) times on each of the tapping points. We suggest about seven times, as you will be repeating a "reminder phrase" while simultaneously tapping, and it may be challenging to be mindful of the number of taps that occurred.

Tapping can occur on either side of the body and, if preferred, both sides can be tapped. It doesn't matter which side is used or whether you alternate between sides during a session. For instance, you can tap under your right eye and then later in the sequence tap under your left arm.

The Points to Tap: Each energy meridian has two end points. You only need to tap on one end to balance out any energy disruptions that may exist. The end points for what Gary Craig refers to as "The Basic Recipe" are near the surface of the body and are therefore more readily accessed than other points along the meridians that may be more deeply located.

The following meridian points of The Sequence are tapped in the order they are presented below (see Figure 11.5):

- At the beginning of the eyebrow, just above and to one side of the nose (EB: Eyebrow).
- On the bone bordering the outside corner of the eye (SE: Side of Eye).
- On the bone under an eye, about one inch below your pupils (UE: Under the Eye).
- Located on the small area between the bottom of your nose and the top of your upper lip (UN: under nose).

■ Midway between the point of your chin and the bottom of your lip (Ch: Chin). Note that this point is not directly on the chin but situated between the chin and the bottom of your lip.

■ The junction where the sternum (breastbone), collarbone, and first rib meet (CB: collar bone). In actuality this point is located just below the collar bone.

■ On the side of the body, at a point even with the nipple (for men) or in the middle of the bra strap for women (UA: under the arm). It is about four inches below the armpit. This area also tends to be sensitive, as it also builds up congestion if it hasn't been rubbed or tapped for some time.

■ For men, one inch below the nipple; for ladies, where the underskin of the breast meets the chest wall (BN: below nipple).

■ On the outside edge of the thumb, at a point even with the base of the thumbnail (Th: thumb).

■ On the side of your index finger (the side closest to your thumb), at a point even with the base of the fingernail (IF: index finger)

■ On the side of your middle finger (the side closest to your thumb), at a point even with the base of the fingernail (MF: middle finger).

■ On the side of your pinky finger (the side closest to your thumb), at a point even with the base of the fingernail (BF: baby finger)

■ The last point is the Karate Chop (KC) point, which has been identified above.

For ease of reference the sequence is listed here:

EB = Beginning of Eyebrow

SE = Side of Eye

UE = Under the Eye

UN = Under the Nose

Ch = Chin

CB = Beginning of the Collarbone

UA = Under the Arm

BN = Below the Nipple

Th = Thumb

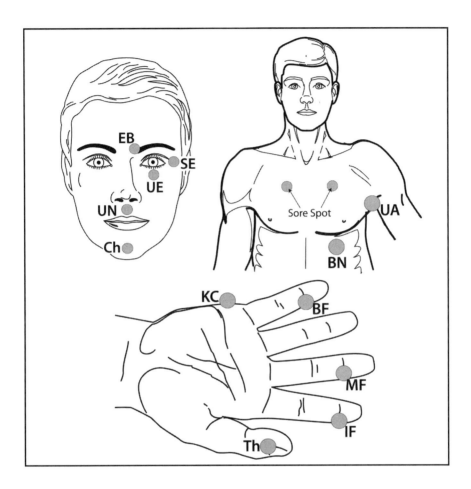

Figure 11.5 Meridian points for the Sequence. Reproduced with permission of the World Center for EFT.

IF = Index Finger

MF = Middle Finger

BF = Baby Finger

KC = Karate Chop

As you have likely noted, the tapping points proceed down the body in an orderly manner, with one tapping point beneath the next.

3. The Nine Gamut Procedure

The Nine Gamut Procedure is without doubt the most bizarre-looking process of all of the EFT procedures, and the one most likely to encounter resistance from your clients. Its purpose is to "fine tune" the brain, which it does through eye movements, humming, and counting. Certain parts of the brain are stimulated through connecting nerves when the eyes are moved. Likewise, the right side of the brain, also known as the nondominant hemisphere (because for most people it does not include language skills), becomes more engaged when you hum a song (Callan et al., 2006; Gunji, Ishii, Chau, Kakigi, & Pantev, 2007; Ozdemir, Norton, & Schlaug, 2006), whereas the left side (dominant hemisphere) is engaged when counting or performing mental calculations of numbers (Ischebeck, Zamarian, Schocke, & Delazer, 2009; Delazer et al., 2003).

The Nine Gamut Procedure is a 10-second process whereby nine of these "brain activating" activities are performed while continuously tapping on one of the body's energy points, namely, the Gamut Point, which must first be located (see Figure 11.6). It is on the back of either hand and is about a half-inch behind the midpoint between the knuckles at the base of the ring and pinky fingers. If you were to draw an imaginary line between the knuckles at the base of the ring and pinky fingers, considering that line as the base of an equilateral triangle whose other sides converge to a point in the direction of the wrist, the gamut point would be located at the apex of this triangle.

Using your first three fingers to tap the flesh area between the two slender bones on the back of your hand (below the pinky and ring finger knuckles) of your opposite hand will surely stimulate the Gamut Point.

Once you've located the Gamut Point, then you are ready to perform nine different actions while simultaneously tapping the GP continuously. They are as follows:

1. Eyes closed.
2. Eyes open.
3. Eyes hard down to the right while holding head still and steady.
4. Eyes hard down to the left while holding head still and steady.
5. Roll eyes in clockwise circular manner as though your nose were the center of a clock and you were trying to see all the numbers.
6. Repeat #5, only in counterclockwise direction.

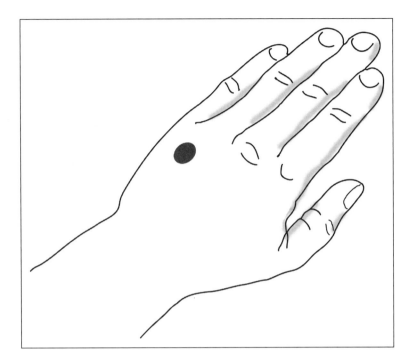

Figure 11.6 The Gamut point.

7. Hum about 2 or 3 seconds of a familiar song ("Happy Birthday" works well).
8. Count rapidly from 1 to 5.
9. Hum another 2 or 3 seconds of a song again.

We recommend that you commit this order to memory and suggest the same for your clients.

4. The Sequence Again

To complete the entire procedure, The Sequence is performed one final time. It may be necessary in some cases to run through steps 3 and 4 more than once to alleviate the presenting concern, but it is generally not necessary to go through all four steps again. In many cases, we find it is only necessary to run through The Sequence again without going through the Nine Gamut Procedure. If one or more repetitions without the PR adjustment are not helpful, including the first step may be necessary, as PR may be the impediment.

At times, we need to remind our clients when going through EFT procedures to "tune in" to the problem they are experiencing. Though this may be emotionally and physically challenging, it is crucial to do so for EFT to be effective. Tuning in simply involves consciously thinking about living with the problem. Unlike what we may do during hypnosis, where we have the person's unconscious mind manifest experiences *without* the problem, during EFT procedures we want the person to dwell on the manifested concern. For habit control work this may mean thinking about smoking a cigarette, or anticipated anxiety about experiencing nicotine withdrawal, or craving a piece of cake, or not exercising. David has personally found EFT to be very beneficial for enhancing the necessary motivation to lace up his shoes and go for a four-to-five mile run. At the same time David has discovered post-exercise EFT to be helpful for managing any physical discomfort, including knee, hip, and ankle pain, after a long run or resistance training session.

THE CASE OF NANCY

As we mentioned previously, Nancy clearly had a bad case of PR that was impeding her ability to lose and keep weight off. She would rebound, or experience "yo-yo"–type weight-loss/weight-gain, like so many well-intentioned dieters. After engaging in a series of muscle-testing exercises and gaining a better understanding of her dilemma with difficulty losing weight, Nancy was willing and ready to pursue EFT, after it was explained to her. Like many of our clients, we forewarn them about what seems to be a series of silly, yet simple procedures that may make them feel just as silly. In many cases, especially when PR is evident, there is little work to do to get a client to try something that might help them. Nancy was no exception.

After learning the procedures, Nancy religiously applied them on a daily basis several times each day, including The PR technique, by rubbing the Sore Spot each time. After asking the four questions mentioned in the previous chapter ("Am I hungry?" "If not, why do I want to eat?" "How will this food make me feel?" and "Will eating this food bring me closer or further away from the trim and fit body I desire?") about why and what she wants to eat and still having a desire to eat, Nancy would go through the EFT procedures, thinking deeply about the cravings she was experiencing. In most situations she was able to curb or completely abate any future cravings. In some situations, even when she continued to crave unhealthy food (usually ice cream), she chose a healthier food instead. She also would start her day off with EFT to help motivate her to go outside for a morning walk that, historically, she had avoided with one excuse or another. In three months, after including EFT in her weight management plan (including Weight Watchers and a diet based on volumetrics, a renewed membership at Curves, and a consistent exercise regimen), Nancy lost 25 pounds. Four months after this she lost an additional 30 pounds, though she had gained 10 pounds in the fifth month after her mother unexpectedly died in a motor vehicle accident. In 1 year, Nancy lost 85 pounds, missing her initial goal by 15 pounds. It was the most weight she had ever lost. For the next 6 months, David saw her twice and during each visit she had maintained her weight loss through a sensible and healthy diet (no longer needing the structure and guidance of Weight Watchers) and regular exercise. She was finding less need to use EFT, as she had developed and internalized a healthy lifestyle without the internal distractions and struggles she had previously experienced.

INTRODUCING TAPPING TO CLIENTS

The process of tapping meridian points may be readily accepted and embraced by some clients. For others it may elicit skepticism and resistance. For those who require a bit more convincing, we suggest the use of analogies and in vivo experiences to heighten their interest and willingness to experiment with Energy Psychology. As with hypnosis, we find it beneficial to establish a "yes set" by asking rhetorical questions that are destined to get a few nods of agreement (Erickson & Rossi, 1979). Muscle testing offers immediate evidence to our clients regarding the direct relationship between thoughts and feelings, and provokes a sense of curiosity about the energy system within the body. Initially, we do not apply energy testing to assess matters like a person's true desire to lose weight (e.g., testing for PR), but we will have our clients answer questions both truthfully and (intentionally) dishonestly, so that they can witness the inherent wisdom within their bodies.

Muscle testing, when done properly, helps a client observe the relationship between their thoughts and feelings and their internal energy system. On the surface we have feelings and behaviors, beneath which lie a set of core beliefs and assumptions that create and drive those feelings and behaviors. Typically, as we explain this to our clients we will get a nod from them, letting us know that they understand and agree with what was just said.

We then address in layman's terms the physiology, biochemistry, and neurology that is fueled by this energy system that they have just seen in action. We explain to them that according to Eastern Medicine philosophy, there is an understanding that the manifestation of illness involves a disruption, distortion, or blockage somewhere within the energy system. We believe this occurs even more so when the problem isn't some somatic pathology, but unhealthy feelings, thoughts, and behaviors. The disruption or blockage in the energy system causes stress, unwanted emotion, or, in habit control work, unwanted urges that promote undesired behavior.

A feedback loop exists between thoughts, feelings, and behaviors that impacts the energy system in either healthy or unhealthy manners. Our thoughts, of course, influence our feelings and behaviors just as our behaviors in turn influence our feelings and thoughts (e.g., guilt/regret for something we did), and our feelings influence our thoughts and behaviors. Any of us with teenage children can attest to the latter, as an adolescent in an irritable mood will dampen the spirits of any party in an instant. Unhealthy thoughts, feelings, or behaviors disrupt the flow of energy which then manifests itself as emotional, mental, and/or physical problems (see Figure 11.7).

With Energy Psychology, or more specifically, EFT procedures described above, the blockages that exist can break, thereby allowing an individual's thoughts, feelings, and behaviors to be healthier, which in turn supports physical, mental, and emotional health and prosperity (see Figure 11.8). We tell our clients that just as a car stereo requires adjustment to more clearly tune in to a channel, so do our bodies require episodic adjustments to permit better and clearer energy flow throughout its system. Introducing EFT will allow a person to enhance energy levels, motivation for change, and optimistic expectations, while reducing physical discomfort, tension, anxiety, negative thought processes, and self-destructive behaviors.

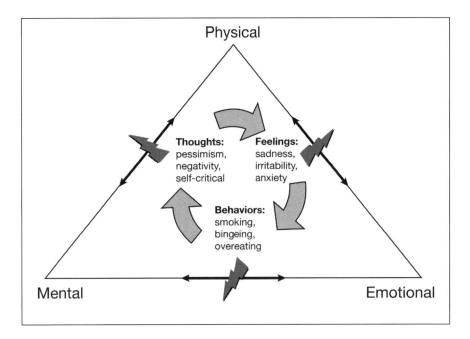

Figure 11.7 Negative energy system.

ENERGY PSYCHOLOGY AND HABIT CONTROL

After applying muscle testing and ensuring consent for treatment, we then ask our clients to identify a particular problem that is occurring at the present moment. Rather than have them identify some future event of concern, we ask them to consider some issue that is present while they are there in the office. We help them identify their problem as concretely and specifically as possible. If they provide us with a response like "I feel really depressed," we seek clarification of that report by asking, "How is it that you feel depressed? What specifically are you experiencing with this depression?" Ultimately, we are seeking concrete responses like "I don't have any energy; I'm just tired all the time" or "I'm angry with my wife" or "My body aches all over." With the latter we may even ask the person to be more specific and select a particular body area that is of most concern. We are not looking for some monumental problem or serious trauma, as we want to ensure success by focusing attention on a more concrete, measurable, or quanti-

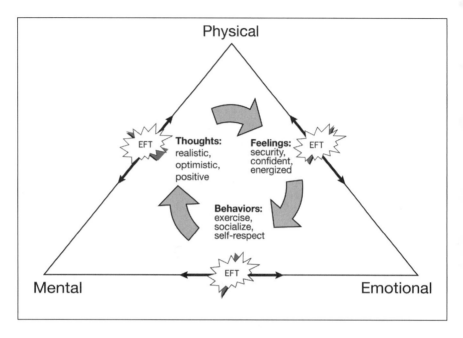

Figure 11.8 Energy system with Emotional Freedom Techniques (EFT).

fiable concern that is relevant to the person right here, right now. If, however, the primary concern lies in the future, that is fine, as we can work with it by having the person recite their affirmative statement in ways that bring it into the present. To do so, we ask them to say, "Even though I am concerned that I will have a craving for ice cream later this evening, I deeply and completely accept myself."

We then have our client rate her concern according to a Subjective Units of Disturbance Scale (SUDS) rating scale ranging from 1 to 10, with 1 being a relatively minor concern and 10 representing overwhelming distress or urges that have become painful and unmanageable. As Energy Psychology relies on positive movement, we want to go beyond the notion of removing what is perceived as negative (e.g., ice cream craving) and help create a more holistic and healthier outcome by installing positive beliefs and cognitions that promote the development of new skills. It is in the development of these new, adaptive skills that we help our clients promote change that becomes permanent.

We may, for instance, ask our client, "How do you want to respond to this situation?" As many clients will frequently provide an answer that involves *moving away* from the temptation (e.g., "I don't want to eat this ice cream; I don't want to be fatter; I don't want this cigarette"), we help reframe those intentions by having them *move toward* something healthy instead. In response to a moving-away-from message, we may say, "But what will you be automatically moving *toward* by not eating this ice cream/not smoking this cigarette? If you weren't feeling bad or feeling fat or feeling like you need to smoke a cigarette, what would you be feeling or doing instead?"

After providing us with an unwanted concern and having completed muscle testing and obtained a SUDS level score, we then introduce the meridian points to the client. We briefly identify each one and do so in the order that they will be tapped. We tap with our clients so that they can mimic us and learn the proper procedures and location of the tapping points. As we are reviewing the points with our clients and they become engaged in the tapping process, it is important to consider that, at this moment, we are actually initiating treatment. Once the client feels comfortable with the process, then we are ready to begin the formal intervention.

We then have the client repeat her affirmation statement as she goes through the procedures, as expanded upon above. As we proceed with the tapping, we have the client repeat the urge or the concern that she can stay focused on, that which is upsetting or distressing. She may say "Urge for a cigarette" or "craving for a piece of cake," or "hip pain," or "very tired." Whatever the concern, it is repeated throughout The Sequence.

Sometimes after the session we learn that a client really resonated with one spot in particular. When this happens we encourage him to use that area to focus on and tap more frequently, or tap again if it seems that this concern has not abated or settled to some extent. We will also offer some suggestions, as we do with hypnosis, to the client while he taps and repeats his "mantra." Using a hypnotic voice, we offer positive suggestions to help the client progress down the path of becoming the permanent nonsmoker or permanently physically fit individual he wants to be: "Notice how your urge can fade, or disappear, as you come even closer to becoming Thomas the permanent non-smoker" or "Just imagine how energized your body will become so that it will be able to resist any urges that take you off the path to becoming the permanently fit and trim Sam you want to be."

When the tapping session is complete, we will ask the client to offer another SUDS score. If it is much lower than the original, then we reinforce the benefits of Energy Psychology and tapping in particular. If the score has changed little, we will go through The Sequence again, with or without the Gamut Procedures (depending upon the client's comfort with the Gamut Procedures) and "fine tune" something that we may have missed. At times, we may need to get our client to be more concrete and specific with their concern. Perhaps the issue is too vague, or the client did not focus adequately on the concern and was instead distracted by making sure he did the procedures correctly. This is not uncommon when people use Energy Psychology for the first time. Going through The Sequence again usually fosters success, as evidenced by a reduced SUDS score.

Potential Problems

At times, you or your client may appreciate limited relief after using Energy Psychology interventions such as tapping. As reported above, in many situations, it is a matter of not having clear, concrete, and specific concerns identified. Sometimes breaking down the concern into its elementary parts can be helpful. For example, a person may report having craved ice cream one evening, yet still desiring not to eat the ice cream, and then actually eating the ice cream after using EFT procedures. During the next session with the client, we may ask her to focus in on what it was about the ice cream that was compelling. Was it the texture, the coolness, the flavor, the sweetness? Perhaps it was emotions or other life challenges that influenced her decision. Consequently, rather than focus on the craving itself, the client could have tended to the emotions she was experiencing at the time. After going through EFT for "craving ice cream," it may have been helpful to use EFT to help with "boredom" or "anger" or "loneliness" or whatever other emotions may have challenged the client from moving down the path of healthier choices.

When we encounter clients who have failed to perceive the benefits of EFT, we always find it helpful to have them run through the EFT procedures to ensure that they are doing them properly. At times, we discover that they either missed steps or were tapping incorrect points or perhaps missing points altogether despite having a handout based on the figures included in this chapter.

After reviewing the procedures with our clients, we will also conduct another session of muscle testing to see if we encounter any PRs. We may discover that results of muscle testing indicate that the client is not motivated to lose weight or stop smoking, and going through the PR intervention may be beneficial for disrupting the energy blockages that serve to frustrate and challenge any benefits of EFT.

Some clients fail to conscientiously focus on the problem and instead consider having the problem dissipate. While we certainly understand that this is the desired reaction, it is important for them to tune in to the problem while going through the tapping procedures.

Below are things to consider for your client in an effort to help her appreciate positive momentum with EFT if she has encountered less than optimal success:

1. Can the client locate the tapping points in order?
2. Does the client tap appropriately? Is the client tapping too hard or too lightly? Is he tapping with three fingers to ensure adequate coverage of the meridian points?
3. Are there any Psychological Reversals interfering with progress? You may need to conduct muscle testing again to adequately rule out this possible impediment to progress.
4. Is the presenting concern specific and concrete? Can it be broken down into more elementary components?
5. Does the client state the concern with appropriate feeling? Is there emotion behind the concern?
6. Is there a particular point that resonates with the client? If so, have the client tap that point while repeating the concern aloud.
7. Did the client repeat the entire procedure or just The Sequence? He may need to run through The Basic Recipe again if the initial SUDS score did not change after EFT.

CONCLUSION

This chapter was exclusively dedicated to a relatively new psychological approach to treating emotional and physical challenges. Energy Psychology borrows interventions and techniques from Eastern Medicine, including acupressure, yoga, qi gong, and energy medicine. It works by stimulating energy points on the surface of the skin, which, when paired with specific psychological procedures, allows a person to change unwanted habits and behaviors. Though there are several procedures used in Energy Psychology for helping people manage unwanted habits, we have found the tapping procedures like those employed with Emotional Freedom Techniques to be the most effective, ecological, and readily applied interventions for helping manage uncomfortable symptoms associated with unwanted behaviors and habits.

We spent a considerable amount of time reviewing the step-by-step procedures of EFT as well as introducing our own spin on tapping meridian points. It has been our experience that despite the apparent simplicity of these techniques, they can provide relief for many symptoms and emotional concerns that may not otherwise receive the relief or respite that the client seeks. While we do encourage our clients to try tapping with any and all problems they encounter, we realize that EFT procedures are not a panacea for severe medical conditions and should never be used in lieu of appropriate medical consultation and care. We would certainly not recommend tapping one's way through a heart attack or stroke or other serious life-threatening medical condition. Nonetheless, our clients have enjoyed the benefits of EFT when applied properly and many maintain that without EFT they might still be smoking or struggling to lose unwanted pounds despite following what seems to be a sensible diet and exercise regimen.

We encourage all practitioners to thoroughly acquaint themselves with Energy Psychology procedures through other readings, videotaped lessons, and workshops and conferences that supplement the information contained in this chapter.

Things to Do

1. Ask a friend or family member to participate in muscle testing. Tell her to answer some questions honestly while intentionally providing false answers to other questions. Note the difference in the resistance of her arm to each question asked.
2. Identify and become familiar with all of the meridian points that are used for tapping. Once you become familiar with the points, go through The Setup, The Sequence, The 9 Gamut Procedures, and The Sequence again. If possible, identify a real-life concern that you are encountering and identify initial and posttreatment SUDS scores.

3. Once you are familiar with the tapping procedures and sequence, introduce them to a friend or family member or, if you feel comfortable doing so, with one of your clients. Again, as we discussed in this chapter, have your client select a very specific, easy-to-identify-and-quantify concern for which EFT has the potential for providing relief. In our experience, when we are not successful with helping a client using Energy Psychology, it is because we did not clearly identify the problem.

12 Putting It All Together

Don't fear failure so much that you refuse to try new things. The saddest summary of a life contains three descriptions: could have, might have, and should have.

—*Louis E. Boone*

We are acutely aware that the effective use of any psychological intervention or combination of interventions such as hypnosis and Energy Psychology involves carefully and strategically tailoring approaches to suit the unique characteristics of each client. We respect and appreciate the individuality of each client who seeks our assistance and service. At the same time, we also recognize the value of modeling as a means of teaching. We have therefore included two extensive case studies in this closing chapter that we hope will help you more capably integrate all of the information and interventions for habit control that have been described throughout this book.

The following case studies involve two clients treated by David in his outpatient clinic. When actual transcripts of the session were available, they have been included. Out of respect for the privacy and confidentiality of both clients, their names, ages, and general background information have been modified to protect their identity, while preserving the accuracy of their presenting concerns.

The first case study involves treatment of a 38-year-old woman named Nancy. You first met Nancy in chapter 11 when we reviewed information on Psychological Reversals and Energy Psychology. The second case study involves treatment of a 23-year-old man named Michael who sought assistance for smoking cessation after 8 years of smoking and multiple efforts to quit, including attendance at a one-session group hypnosis intervention that was "guaranteed" to help all participants kick the habit.

THE CASE OF NANCY

Background Information

Nancy was 38 years old at the time she first sought treatment with David. She stood 5 feet, 7 inches tall and weighed 235 pounds, resulting in a BMI of 36.8, which is well into the obesity range. She had been divorced for 3 years after 6 years of marriage and had no children. Her separation and divorce was rather amicable, as she and her former husband had little in common and recognized that they would each be better off pursuing relations with other people.

Nancy had been employed for the last 6 years as a line worker at the local Hershey's Chocolate plant. She enjoyed her job, worked overtime whenever opportunities to do so were available, yet she was concerned that the physical demands of her job were compromising her physical well-being, particularly her knees and back. She had consulted an orthopedic surgeon, who recommended a double knee replacement, though he informed her that she might be able to avoid invasive surgery if she lost about 70 pounds.

Complicating matters, Nancy also suffered from type 2 diabetes mellitus, hypertension, and chronic obstructive pulmonary disease. Her knee and back pain precluded regular exercise, though she did try to walk twice weekly when pain was limited; she also swam at the local physical fitness center at least three times a week. She had been trying to lose weight throughout most of her adult life, though her history generally involved losing no more than 20 pounds only to see it return within a matter of months. She tried Curves, Weight Watchers, the South Beach Diet, and The Atkins Diet, all without any prolonged success.

Nancy did not struggle with weight issues as a young child. She reported being a healthy and very active youngster who played field hockey and soccer in high school. After moving out of her parents' home and getting married, she became reclusive, isolative, and tended to sit at home with her husband who was never a physically active individual. Though she wanted children, her husband did not. When she wasn't putting in extra hours at Hershey's, she was at home watching television with her husband. She frequently dined on carry-out meals from drive-thru fast-food establishments before heading home. Though Nancy had played sports in high school, she was never an avid exerciser because playing sports itself enabled her to stay fit. Over the past 8 to 10 years, Nancy gained nearly 110 pounds and felt horrible about herself.

After her divorce, she remained isolated, feeling that she wasn't worthy to date anyone, given her physical appearance and condition. It didn't really help matters that she worked at a candy factory where she was able to purchase Reese's Pieces and Peanut Butter Cups at a discounted rate, which she took advantage of quite frequently.

Session 1

During the initial interview it was readily apparent that Nancy used a good bit of "past talk." She would frequently refer to her life failings (no children) and reflect on past losses (e.g., her marriage). Her language was very pessimistic and negative; she would frequently offer excuses as to why she wasn't able to lose weight and keep it off. Despite telling David that she has "tried all the diets out there," it became apparent after further questioning that Nancy tended to sabotage her diets by eating unhealthy between-meal snacks like Reese's Pieces and Peanut Butter Cups. She also had a "sweet tooth" for mint chocolate chip ice cream.

Nancy went on very few dates during high school, as she was focused on playing sports throughout the year. Consequently her level of confidence about dating was very poor and hampered by her limited experiences and body image. Her longest relationship was with her husband and she perceived that as a failed relationship, owing to her own insecurities and dependency.

During the initial habit assessment, Nancy reported being a stress eater who binged after coming home from work and sat alone while watching television. When consciously considering her choice of unhealthy foods, she reported "feeling sorry for myself" and having a general attitude that binging on candy and ice cream "really didn't matter because no one would want to be with me anyway." After losing 20 pounds, she generally found it difficult to continue to adhere to her diet, as it became physically uncomfortable to restrict her daily consumption. She also found that she "missed" her ice cream, which she perceived as "a friend who could comfort me when I was feeling bad."

Session 2

Nancy completed the Locus of Control Scale and RHETI sampler after her first session. Her resultant score of 23 on the Rotter Scale was indicative of an individual with an extreme external locus of control. In essence, Nancy maintained that she had limited control over her destiny, which may challenge therapeutic progress and consequently will need to be addressed at some time during her treatment.

Results of the RHETI sampler indicated that she was either a Type Two (Helper) or Type Six (Loyalist). Given the equivocal findings, she took the online version of the full RHETI, which revealed that she was a Type Six with a Seven-wing. Recall from chapter 3 that Sixes are best known for being committed. They are engaging, responsible, anxious, and suspicious, and maintain a basic fear that they will be alone without support and guidance. Sixes are generally known to be hard working, reliable, vigilant, persevering, cautious, and anxious. They can be pessimistic, doubtful, negativistic and reactive and at their worst may be suspicious and blaming. Nancy's workaholic personality and underlying anxiety and dependency support findings from the Enneagram. You will also recall that Sixes tend to stew in a state of anxiety. Even if there is nothing to worry about, Sixes will surely find something to worry about.

Because well-functioning Sixes look like Healthy Nines, one goal of therapy would be to help Nancy become more engaging, playful, friendly, and understanding and accepting of life's ups and downs. It was apparent from the initial contact that David was going to have to address Nancy's general sense of insecurity and help her understand that security comes from within. Knowing that Nancy was quite capable of supporting herself financially, taking care of her bills, and being a responsible citizen, David could capitalize on these strengths and use this evidence of self-sufficiency to help Nancy minimize her anxiety and fear of things she could not control or predict in her life.

Given her sense of loyalty, David also understood that Nancy would function best by seeking others or joining a group of people who share a common goal like losing weight or becoming permanently fit and trim. Exercising with others, attending health-focused seminars, and joining a gym could be very therapeutic for Nancy, but recommending this would likely stand a greater chance of acceptance after a few sessions. David would first need to address Nancy's insecurities and anxieties, as she was not prepared to engage with others. She would likely need to lose some weight and witness some success and confidence before feeling comfortable enough to participate in group activities.

Sixes, like Fives also benefit from information, though overload and inconsistent data could generate additional anxiety, which must be minimized—or avoided, if at all possible. Therefore, providing Sixes with "just the facts" that can be readily backed up and supported by some expert documentation could be helpful.

Sixes can also be rather indecisive and are prone to "yes, but" themselves, as they fear making commitments. Hypnotherapy sessions that include self-affirming statements as well as opportunities to image and create success can reinforce a self-support system that Nancy desperately requires if she is to continue to realign her identity as an individual committed to a lifestyle that is reflective of a person who is fit and healthy.

After reviewing results from the Rotter Scale and the Enneagram during the second session, David provided Nancy with some focused information on weight management and diabetes and recommended that she purchase a recipe book that relied on volumetrics to enhance weight loss. She indicated that she found some success in the past using Weight Watchers and planned to reinitiate this diet later in the week. David supported this, but informed her that "temporary diets" that are not intended to be part of her daily lifestyle are likely doomed to failure at some point in the future. He also encouraged her to keep a daily food diary so that they could review her food choices and address some of the underlying reasons supporting her unhealthy eating habits. Finally, David and Nancy agreed upon a moderate exercise regimen, endorsed by her physician, that consisted of 20-minute walks around her neighborhood three times weekly in addition to an anaerobic resistance training program (consisting of pyramiding and muscle isolation exercises) twice weekly. In addition to this, she could swim as many days during the week as she would like, but she was not to substitute swimming for walking. Though swimming is an excellent means of cardiovascular exercise, its weight loss benefits are limited. Finally, Nancy was encouraged to consult a specialized shoe store to ensure that she was wearing a shoe that was ideal for her, as it was apparent from looking at the bottom of her shoes that she tended to pronate when walking. She also had a very high arch that would likely require support to minimize hip and knee pain.

Session 3

Nancy brought her daily diet diary to her third session. A sampling of her weekly diet is listed in Table 12.1.

Based on the three days' daily diet diary, it is readily apparent that Nancy was having difficulties moderating her food consumption. Based on her age, weight, height, and daily activity level (relatively sedentary), Nancy could consume up to 2,239 calories per day and break even. Essentially, if she was not exercising at all she could consume 2,239 calories per day and would not gain weight. If she engaged in light activities requiring some but limited physical effort during the day, she could consume an additional 100 calories per day, while exercising regularly would permit her to consume nearly 3,000 calories per day before she would gain any weight. As can be determined from the numbers above, based on the sampling of her daily caloric intake, Nancy was consuming between 500 and 1,500 extra calories per day, which of course will lead to increased weight gain.

Fortunately, as well as can be determined, Nancy was likely providing accurate data regarding her daily diet. At times, clients may be less than forthcoming with their dietary habits, tending to minimize the bad while reporting the good. When seeing reports that are "too good to be true," especially when there is weight gain and not weight loss, we encourage our clients to reconsider their report, reflect upon the last week, and see if they left out any between-meal snacks or "extra helpings" that weren't reported. In most cases, we find our clients then "correct" their daily diary, thereby making sense of their struggles to lose weight.

Knowing that Nancy needed to make adjustments not only to what but how she ate, David asked Nancy to consider the Four Questions reviewed in the Mindfulness chapter (chapter 10). She was asked to consider these questions each time she was thinking of eating. To help her with these questions, Nancy posted the list on her refrigerator in large red letters:

- Question #1: Am I hungry?
- Question #2: If I am not hungry, why do I want to eat?
- Question #3: How will eating this food make me feel, emotionally and physically, immediately after eating it, 2 minutes from now, 10 minutes from now, and 30 minutes from now?

Table 12.1

Sampling of Nancy's Weekly Diet

Day/Time	Food	Quantity	Calories	Emotions/Context	Hungry?	Result
Sunday 7 am	Weight Watcher's applesauce pancakes, turkey bacon, English muffin with butter, apple juice	Medium	690	None. First meal of the day.	Yes	Satiated.
9:30 am	10 Ginger snaps	Medium	200	Bored; a little anxious.	Slight	Still bored.
12 pm	Lean pockets stuffed sandwich, low fat potato chips, diet soda	Medium	360	Alone, time for lunch, ate too fast.	Yes!	Satiated, but ate too many chips—a little guilty about that.
2:15 pm	3 scoops MC-chip ice cream	Large	360	Bored, ate one scoop, which led to two more.	Slightly	Angry at self.
6:30 pm	Weight Watchers chicken enchiladas, steamed vegetables	Medium	300	Very hungry.	Yes	Better.
11:45 pm	Three packs of peanut butter cups	Medium	780	Watching TV, saw commercial of couple going on vacation, became sad.	Not really	Sad and angry.
2:30 am	One pack of peanut butter cups, glass of whole milk	Small	390	Woke up, couldn't get back to sleep, worried about nothing in particular, just an internal feeling.	Not sure	Tired.

DAILY CALORIC INTAKE: 2780

(continued)

Table 12.1 *(continued)*

Day/Time	Food	Quantity	Calories	Emotions/Context	Hungry?	Result
Tuesday 6:30 am	English muffin with peanut butter, glass of whole milk, 2 bowls of granola cereal	Medium	740	First meal of the day before going to work.	Yes	Satiated.
9:50 am	Two packages of Peanut butter cups, one bag of Reese's Pieces, Diet Coke	Medium	670	Break at work.	Some	Disappointed.
12:30 pm	Lean pockets stuffed sandwich, bag of low fat potato chips, package of Oreos from vending machine, Diet Coke	Medium	470	Lunch at work with colleagues, saw friend eating cookies so I bought some. Thought "won't matter."	Yes	Satiated, but upset about eating cookies.
2:40 pm	Bag of Reese's Pieces	Small	210	Break, had bag of Reese's Pieces in my purse.	Slightly	Kind of numb.
6:00 pm	Weight Watchers glazed chicken frozen dinner, steamed vegetables	Medium	210	Very hungry.	Yes	Still hungry.
7:00 pm	Weight Watcher's lean pocket stuffed sandwich	Medium	260	Watching TV, still hungry after dinner.	Yes	Satiated, feel okay with good choice for food.
10:50pm	Two scoops of MCC ice cream, with chocolate sauce	Medium	580	Wanted to eat something; feeling anxious while watching television.	A little	Some anxiety, not sure why, wanted to eat more but didn't.

DAILY CALORIC INTAKE: 3140

Table 12.1 (*continued*)

Day/Time	Food	Quantity	Calories	Emotions/Context	Hungry?	Result
Wednesday 6:45 am	English muffin with peanut butter, glass of whole milk, 2 hard-boiled eggs	Medium	625	First meal of the day before going to work.	Yes	Satiated.
9:30 am	Two packages of Pea-nut butter cups	Medium	480	Break at work.	Some	Still hungry.
10:00 am	Package of pretzels from vending machine	Small	230	Needing snack.	Yes	More comfortable, but craving some-thing sweet.
12:40 pm	Ordered McDonald's with coworkers: Quarter Pounder with Cheese, Large Fries, Apple Pie, Diet Coke	Large	1320	Lunch—coworker going to McDon-ald's offered to pick up meal. Didn't have time to pack lunch that morning due to making breakfast. Very hungry.	Yes	Very full, heart rate increased, felt bad physically. Upset with self for eating fast food, though "got over it" by end of work day.
6:00 pm	Weight Watchers glazed chicken frozen dinner, steamed vege-tables	Medium	210	Very hungry.	Yes	Still hungry—like the night before, this wasn't enough to eat.
7:00 pm	Nachos with cheese, olives, nacho sauce	Medium	370	Watching TV, still hungry after din-ner.	Yes	Satiated, feel okay with choice for food—could have been worse.
10:30 pm	Dairy Queen Blizzard	Medium	580	Feeling anxious, not sure why.	A little	Sick, anxious and worried, went to bed upset, cried.

DAILY CALORIC INTAKE: 3815

■ Question #4: Will eating this food in this amount move me closer to or further away from becoming the permanently slim and fit person I want to be?

Asking these questions did indeed adjust her dietary habits, as she frequently refrained from eating, particularly when she realized that she wasn't hungry. Unfortunately, there was little carry-over at work and she continued to eat Reese's Pieces and Peanut Butter Cups on an almost daily basis. She was able to report that in the evening anxiety seemed to worsen and triggered her unhealthy diet choices and episodic overeating.

Session 4

David introduced the concept of hypnosis to Nancy during their first session and revisited it during the fourth session. She was very open to the opportunity and in fact had sought out David's services after seeing a brochure for one of his group therapy programs for weight management. Unfortunately, due to limited interest, David was unable to get this group going. Consequently, after meeting with Nancy, he offered her the opportunity to work with him individually. She had no preconceived notion that hypnosis would offer a quick and easy fix to her weight problem, though like most people she had very little experience or understanding about hypnosis. After David explained the procedures, employing presupposition and utilization techniques (based on Nancy's history of playing sports and the piano), Nancy was eager to get started. Through hypnosis, David was hoping to enable Nancy to get in touch with a "future self" who was motivated and dedicated to becoming permanently fit and trim. Additionally, hypnosis could promote a sense of self-acceptance that Nancy lacked. Hypnosis could also be used to help manage her pain and physical discomfort, which at times precluded her from engaging in exercise. Finally, knowing that Nancy has not had a life-long battle with her weight, David could utilize hypnosis to help Nancy get in touch with her athletic, healthy, physically active self that still possesses skills and resources that can be mobilized in the present.

The following are excerpts from one of David's hypnosis sessions. When appropriate, we have included bracketed personal commentary about strategies and interventions that were employed. The session began after David invited Nancy to sit in a recliner (her preference), turned the lights down, closed the blinds, and turned off his cell phone. All of these modifications serve as contextual cues for clients to prepare for trance. Over time, with enough experience, these contextual cues allow clients to initiate trance before the therapist begins any "formal" verbal induction techniques.

> Okay Nancy, just make yourself as comfortable as you can be. [It is not necessary for clients to be completely comfortable for trance to occur (just consider the waking trance we experience while driving a car), which is why we encourage them to be *as comfortable as possible*.] If you want, you can take a slow deep breath in through your nose…and gently release through your mouth…you can do that a few times to help you settle…allow your conscious mind to quiet…to take a time-out, so your unconscious mind can be more available to you now…that's right [reinforcing her behavior as she follows the suggestion]. Just allow your mind to wander…or to settle [it will do one or the other so this directive promotes a win–win situation]…with each breath you take, you can imagine how the oxygen you take in heals and sooths every cell of your body…allowing every muscle to become more comfortable…setting the stage for you to *go into trance* [these words are timed and spoken as Nancy exhales]…and with each breath you exhale…you can imagine all the stress and tension you've been holding becoming released and let go…so each breath out releases any uncomfortable feeling, freeing your mind…to *go into trance*…and with each breath you may begin to feel yourself *go into trance* in a way that is comfortable for you (Nancy adjusts herself in the recliner; pushing herself back)…and any time you need to adjust yourself…to help you *go into trance* is fine…we know the more comfortable we feel the easier it is to *go into trance*…and *stay in trance*…this is just an opportunity for you to get in touch with skills and resources…resources that are there *deep within you* [again timed with her breathing, with an emphasis on the word "deep" to subtly enhance her trance]…you may even notice that your body begins to feel different as you *go into trance*; like going into a pool…you can decide how much *deeper* you want to go…you can always find a comfortable place to be and stay right there in that *comfortable trance state*…or, if you want like that person in a pool, *go all the way in*…it really doesn't matter…it's really up to you [giving the client control of their trance, in our experience, creates a greater opportunity for trance to occur]…there are many ways you can *go into trance*…realize your body and mind have had a lot of experience going *into trance*…when you played sports I'm sure there were times you found yourself in that…*zone*…that place where you just let your body do what you knew it could do. Just *letting go*…trusting that your body knew what to do…or like when you play the piano…there's no need to think about every key stroke you're about to make…your mind and body work together to just *allow it to happen*…it's natural and familiar…and just like that you can *go into trance*…now…taking the time now to get in touch with the Nancy who was *active…fit…trim…*energized…knowing that your unconscious mind can still access all that was there…like calling up a memory triggered by an image…or a scent…like smelling Play Doh or Silly

Putty takes you back to a time and place when you were a young child...it remembers...it knows and can help you now...and later [planting the seeds for future success]...and if you want to go *deeper* into trance, you can get in touch with all of those resources...the more comfortable you feel...maybe you can even notice how *different* you feel now than you did when you first came into my office today...noticing that difference and how your unconscious mind helps this trance, this opportunity [using the principle of Linking to enhance her trance experience]...and like the athlete preparing for competition...imagining *success*...seeing herself where she wants to be...doing what she wants to do...and like that you can see yourself...the permanently slim and fit Nancy...seeing yourself in a place and time where you look and feel and move around as the *permanently slim and fit* Nancy... like a movie that fast forwards into the future...as days pass...as images of days on a calendar are ripped off and tossed away...you can see the size of your clothing *going down*...seeing the numbers on the scale *going down*... imagine how you feel...how others notice the changes you've made...making comments about how you look...how you eat...asking how you *lost that weight*...maybe you can even see yourself making good choices about what you eat...seeing how easy it is to say *no to that ice cream*...say *no to those Reese's peanut butter cups*...knowing to say no brings you closer to the permanently slim and fit Nancy you want to be...with each breath you exhale, imagine how you will feel as the permanently slim, fit, healthy Nancy [more linking]...see how well you move...how freely you move...how *comfortably you move* [subtle wording suggesting the absence of pain without specifically stating it]...I invite you now to take some time while I remain silent...time to just imagine whatever you want to imagine...think what you want to think...just letting your unconscious mind mobilize and access that which is within...to help you now...and later...I will now be quiet for about two minutes of clock time and when I start talking again you can continue to be comfortable...to stay in trance [presupposition that she is in trance] before you need to be more alert and oriented to an awake state. (Two minutes of silence pass). Very good...just continue to be comfortable...to allow your unconscious mind to take all of this experience in...to make it part of you...part of your experience...imagining how you can do that...maybe like a sponge absorbs water...taking it in...or just filing it away somewhere in your mind...somewhere that it becomes available for you when you need it...some place safe but available. (She takes in a noticeably deeper breath)...that's right...just take this experience in...make it part of who you are...part of the permanently slim and fit Nancy that you know you can be. So when you are ready...when you feel you have internalized this experience...when you feel that it is part of you and there for you...then you can begin to be more alert...come back to the here and now place in my office [more presupposition that a trance occurred, something has been internalized, and trance is concluding], move or stretch your arms and legs...gently open your eyes so that you can become familiar with the lighting in the room as it may be brighter in here than you remember. (Nancy stretches her arms above her head, slowly opens her eyes and stares at the ceiling)…very good…welcome back…when you're ready to talk, let me know how that went for you [this invitation allows the client to come out of trance gently, as some people are not immediately prepared to talk].

Session 5

Nancy reported that she lost 6 pounds in the past 2 weeks. She began walking twice weekly and had purchased some dumbbells of varying weights which she was using three times weekly, mostly for her upper body. She began employing the pyramid principle and though her shoulders and arms were sore for a few days after her first weight training session, later in the first week she felt well enough to lift again and had done so four times since the last session. Nancy also informed David that she had not eaten any Reese's Peanut Butter Cups or Reese's Pieces during the last week. When asked what helped her not eat this candy, she reported that "I just didn't want it. I knew that it wasn't going to help me lose weight and that it really did matter if I ate them." She had one bowl of ice cream during the week, and otherwise, followed her Weight Watcher's diet.

The remainder of the fifth session was dedicated to more hypnosis. During hypnosis, David continued to focus on helping Nancy create a path leading to the future self she desired, helping her make connections between her decisions and the permanently slim and fit person she wanted to be. This also required helping her gain greater control over her internalized anxiety. Though Nancy had never suffered from panic attacks, David's approach during hypnosis was very much like what he would do with individuals suffering from episodes of uncontrollable panic. Using the Class of Problems/Class of Solutions model, David considered *how* a person makes a panic attack, with the understanding that people "make" panic attacks by internalizing emotions, initiating a fight-or-flight reaction, creating adrenaline and cortisol to make the heart race faster and turn off the parasympathetic nervous system while turning on the sympathetic nervous system. For Nancy, the problem is anxiety and the class of problems is characterized as uncontrolled fight-or-flight phenomenon. The way to control fight-or-flight (or minimize the impact of the sympathetic nervous system) is to enhance the parasympathetic system response, which is accomplished through rest and relaxation. As we mentioned in a prior chapter (chapter 9 on Ericksonian hypnosis), panic and anxiety are essentially the result of the autonomic nervous system gone awry. Through trance, David used suggestions that facilitated and elicited a relaxation response automatically versus that which was under conscious control. As we mentioned earlier, trance works best for concerns that are involuntary and, for Nancy, her anxiety felt very much out of her control.

Over time, Nancy was reporting less anxiety and fewer incidents of eating unhealthy food that was triggered by anxiety and boredom.

Session 6

Nancy lost 8 more pounds during the seventh week of treatment. She had lost a total of 14 pounds since initiating treatment and was maintaining very good momentum, which was reinforced in trance during this session. Nancy continued to make good dietary choices and purchased a book recommended by David that established a diet based on volumetrics. She reported that the recipes were easy to follow and the meals were "very filling and actually tasty." She also continued to eat Weight Watchers meals but was no longer monitoring the points of this program.

David had Nancy bring in her weekly diet diary, which she continued to maintain, and it was clearly a healthier diet with fewer episodes of anxiety reported. She indicated that during the evenings, rather than watching television and feeling anxious, she had been going to a gym three times weekly, where she met other women who were planning to exercise together. She continued to work any and all overtime opportunities at the factory, though she was not seeing this as escapism or a means of managing her anxiety. She had not been spending any money at the vending machine and still had not eaten any of the candy that had become a staple of her diet.

During her hypnosis session, David emphasized her progress to date, using images and metaphors that underscored her progress to date. For example, he mentioned the life examples of famous athletes who encountered significant obstacles that appeared to be career-ending but weren't, as the athlete continued to maintain a sense of accomplishment in his sport and a desire to once again play and be at the top of his game. During this session he asked Nancy to reflect on her own life experience as "perhaps there is something there in your past where you had to work hard, to move yourself forward, to take small steps that eventually lead to bigger steps." After this session Nancy shared an incident where she had torn a calf muscle and was sidelined from playing field hockey for several weeks. During that time she became depressed and isolated, even from her teammates. After a few days of wallowing in self-pity she recognized that this was doing her no good and that her true desire was to play at least one more game before the season ended. With the assistance of a physical therapist, Nancy was able to rehabilitate her injury and six weeks after being injured played in a game, scoring two goals. She played in two more games before the season ended, and though she didn't score any more goals, felt very good about her accomplishments and ability to meet and exceed her goal of playing in at least one more game before the season ended.

Nancy's homework for the week was to continue with her exercise program and continue with her diet, which was becoming a lifestyle rather than a means to an end. She had been finding success with socializing with others because of her involvement at the local fitness center, and she was indeed looking more like a healthy Nine rather than an unhealthy Six.

Session 7

Nancy reported losing four more pounds, but was disappointed that she did not lose more weight. She had noticed that with each week that passed, she was able to lose more weight than she had the week before. During the middle of the week, she had only lost 2 pounds and became somewhat distressed. The following day, rather than become motivated to exercise, she stayed home, watched television, and ate two bowls of ice cream. Though she knew that she was engaging in self-sabotaging behavior, she reported that she "couldn't help it." She sensed that she was on the path to self-destruction and had even told herself that she just wasn't capable of losing any more than 20 pounds since she hadn't done it before.

David and Nancy spent half of this session reviewing her week and examining where things went wrong as well as examining where things had been going right. Focusing on her successes over the past several weeks was helpful for gaining the momentum and motivation that she needed to stay the course. Hypnosis was deferred for this session and David introduced Nancy to EFT (Emotional Freedom Techniques). As reported above, during muscle testing Nancy displayed Psychological Reversal regarding her desire to lose weight. Though she was initially very distressed to learn that her body was telling her she did not want to lose weight while her mind believed something different, going through the Energy Psychology procedures helped undo the Psychological Reversal that was perhaps impacting her progress, at least during the past week.

Nancy embraced the notion of Energy Psychology and the EFT techniques with tapping. She readily identified the meridian points and prior to the conclusion of this session was able to go through the entire procedure. Nancy did not, however, utilize the Nine Gamut Procedure and instead relied upon The Sequence during this session and following weeks. She was encouraged to use the procedures whenever she had cravings to eat candy or ice cream, when feeling anxious or bored, or during any situation in which she felt uncomfortable or in pain. She was also encouraged to identify pre- and post-SUDS (Subjective Units of Disturbance Scale) scores and record them.

Session 8

Nancy arrived for this session in very good spirits. She reported losing only 4 more pounds during the past week, however her total weight loss to date was 22 pounds "and counting," as she said. She was thrilled that she had finally lost more than 20 pounds and appeared to continue to be losing weight. Her average daily caloric intake was about 1,800 calories. She was still exercising and reported that, though she continued to experience knee and back pain, it was reduced to the extent that she was able to continue walking. She had started swimming again this week, though had not changed her regimen otherwise.

She had been using the EFT procedures during the week and found them beneficial for minimizing anxiety in the evening and managing pain after exercise. Her SUDS scores in most cases dropped 4 to 5 points after tapping. There were times, however, when her scores didn't change despite repeated tapping and revisions to her tapping that reflected more concrete and specific focus on concerns.

The last half of this session was dedicated to hypnosis, which continued to reinforce the permanence of her habit control and minimize her experienced anxiety. David continued to include visualizations of a future Nancy, vividly experiencing herself having the body she desired, living in this body and interacting with others who recognize and comment on this permanently fit and trim Nancy.

Session 9

It had been 2 weeks since David last saw Nancy, as he was out of town and unable to meet with her for their regularly scheduled visit. It had been 12 weeks since their initial visit and Nancy had lost three more pounds for a total of 25 pounds to date. She did report "cheating" some days by eating ice cream, and on two occasions grabbing dinner at a fast food drive-thru. She offered no excuses other than being hungry and in a hurry on those 2 days. She realized that there would be good days and bad days, and, rather than become anxious or self-degrading about the matter, she was beginning to "go with the flow" a bit more readily.

Session 10

This was Nancy's last weekly appointment. She and David agreed that, if she was making good progress and beginning to internalize new and healthier habits that became part of her lifestyle, weekly sessions would no longer be necessary and monthly follow-up appointments could ensue. During this session Nancy and David reviewed her progress to date and spent the last half of the session doing hypnosis. David made a CD audio recording for Nancy to use at home until they met again in one month. The recording was a relatively generic hypnosis session that reinforced much of what had already been established during prior sessions and emphasized her positive attributes, provided suggestions for relaxation and comfort, and again offered the opportunity for Nancy to allow her subconscious mind to set the stage for perceiving the permanently slim and fit Nancy.

Session 11

Nancy returned to David's office for her first follow-up appointment about five weeks after their last session. She reported losing another 10 pounds. Her total weight loss since initiating treatment about four months prior to this visit was 35 pounds. She was very pleased with her progress, and friends and some family members were beginning to compliment her on her weight loss. Her youngest sister, however, remained rather critical, though Nancy took this in stride. Initially she was very upset that her sister made comments like, "This isn't any different than any other time you've lost weight. You lose it and gain it right back." Fortunately Nancy knew her sister was incorrect about her assumption. Nancy hadn't tried to lose weight by doing all that she was now doing. She was focused on making this a permanent adjustment in her life, a lifestyle change that would promote continued success.

All other matters in her life were rather settled and she reported that she continued to work at Hershey's, taking whatever hours she could get. She had considered looking for another job, given some of the episodic temptations she had with purchasing candy from the factory, though at least up until this time she hadn't done so.

Nancy was still using the EFT procedures, though not as frequently. She had listened to the CD David made for her a few times each week, but was finding that her dietary changes and exercise regimen were becoming a natural part of her life and were allowing her to continue to lose weight and move down the path to becoming the Nancy she wanted to be with the body she wanted to have. She and David agreed to meet in one to two months for a follow-up, with plans of discontinuing services soon after that if all was still going well.

Session 12

It had been 6 weeks since her last visit, and 10 days ago Nancy's mother died unexpectedly from traumatic injuries sustained in a motor vehicle accident. Up to that point in time, Nancy was doing very well. She lost an additional 10 pounds, but gained it right back after her mother's death. Initially, Nancy became isolative, sleeping through the day, eating little to nothing. Within 4 days after her mother's funeral, she began to overeat and consume very unhealthy foods. She had little to no energy to prepare her own meals, and though she had become very interested and inspired in cooking her own meals, she was no longer interested in going into the kitchen unless it was to retrieve some ice cream.

Fortunately, as she began to notice her weight gain, she was able to ward off any further emotional decline after some of the friends she met at the fitness center began calling her and picking her up so that she would exercise with them. Though initially reluctant to join them, she found it difficult to resist their invitation when three of them arrived at her front door and waited for her to change into her sweats before they drove her to the gym. The workout was difficult and energy-draining, though she felt better for having done it. The next day she went for a walk and after meeting with David had decided that her mother would not want her to give up on herself, given the progress that she had made thus far. She became rather steadfast in getting into better shape and maintaining a healthy lifestyle "for her mother." At least for the following few months, that was the driving impetus to go to the gym, or go for a walk, or make sure she ate healthy meals and snacks through the day.

She assured David that she would be okay and that she would continue to dedicate her life to the permanently slim and healthy Nancy that she was readily becoming. David informed her that if she was able to maintain this healthy lifestyle after such a traumatic and upsetting experience, that there would be little to deter her in the future. This setback showed Nancy that she was truly dedicated to herself and the body that she desired.

Session 13

Nancy met with David 6 weeks after their last visit and had lost an additional 15 pounds. The visit was cut short, as she had to attend a job interview an hour later. She reported that she was doing very well and it was apparent that she continued to lose weight and her self-confidence had improved tremendously. She was applying for a job as a receptionist in a dentist's office and, though she had no experience as a receptionist, had been taking some online computer courses and had familiarized herself with a number of word-processing programs. She had engaged in more social activities than she ever had before and though she was still not dating anyone that was fine with her. She had a number of opportunities to go out on dates with a number of different men, however, she didn't feel that she was quite ready for this yet.

She hadn't used EFT procedures nor listened to the hypnosis CD since last seeing David and didn't think that any of it was necessary. She told David that she knew that these resources were available for her should she need them and this allowed her to have an even greater level of confidence about herself that was not present before. Once each week, she would allow herself to eat something that was "less than ideal," including some ice cream, but she found the following day she was ready to continue with the lifestyle that she was consciously choosing that helped her lose weight. Some days she opted not to "treat" herself.

Her pain had been more manageable since losing nearly 50 pounds. She was hoping to lose another 50 pounds in 4 months, as her goal was to lose 100 pounds in 1 year, though she was prepared to "be okay" with this if she fell short of her goal.

Though she and David believed that subsequent sessions were no longer indicated at this time, she agreed to return to his office in three months to provide an updated report and determine if subsequent treatment was needed. David encouraged Nancy to contact him at any time should she require any assistance, and three months went by without a call from her.

Session 14

One week shy of 1 year and Nancy had lost 85 pounds. She lost an additional 30 pounds in the past 4 months, and though she was 15 pounds shy of her established goal of 100 pounds, she was very pleased with her progress, and very confident that she would be able to shed 15 pounds in the next few months. She wanted to try some more hypnosis during this session, as she was finding that some anxiety crept back into her life since starting a new job at a veterinarian's office. She didn't get the job at the dentist's office, but a friend who was a veterinary assistant told her about a job that was opening at her office and, after applying and interviewing with two of the practice's owners, Nancy was offered the job. She had regular hours, better pay, good benefits that were comparable to what she had at Hershey, though she was finding it difficult at times to deal with some impatient and demanding clients.

David discussed these concerns with her and offered her the opportunity to come back for regular weekly visits; she declined, believing that she would be able to adequately handle things before they "got out of control." She was sleeping without difficulty and was maintaining a very sensible diet and exercise regimen, though there had been some days when she found it difficult to get to the gym, especially on weekends.

THE CASE OF MICHAEL

Background Information

Michael was a 23-year-old Caucasian male who was referred to David by his primary care physician for smoking cessation. Michael reported smoking about one to one-and-a-half packs of cigarettes per day for the past 5 years. Prior to that, he smoked less than a pack a day, though indicated he had a desire to smoke more often but was restricted by his mother, who forbade him to smoke in her home. He had started smoking when a friend stole a pack of his mother's cigarettes and the two of them smoked after school. Over time, he found other friends to smoke with and by the time he was 16 years old Michael was smoking over a half-pack each day. At the time of the initial consultation, Michael was living with his girlfriend of 2 years, Sharon, who was a nonsmoker. Since moving in together 6 months ago, Sharon has "pestered" him to quit smoking. He attended a one-session stop-smoking program using hypnosis; however, he found this program to be of little benefit, as he smoked two cigarettes while driving home after the program.

Michael was an only child, raised by his mother. He never knew his father, as his birth was the result of a "one-night-stand" and his mother chose to raise him on her own. Though Michael reports that at times he would like to have known his father, or have the option to attempt to locate him, he did report understanding his mother's predicament and reasons behind her decision to keep this information from him.

His psychiatric history was noncontributory, though his family physician did prescribe Wellbutrin to assist with smoking cessation. In general, Michael was opposed to medication and informed David during their first session that he had no interest in trying Chantix.

His medical history was contributory for tonsillectomy at age 18 and, over the course of the past few months before meeting David, he suffered from a number of colds that tended to linger longer than usual. He was not taking any prescriptive or over-the-counter medication. He was a high school graduate who attended tech school and had been employed as a heating and air conditioning technician for the past 18 months. Prior to that, he worked as a stock clerk in a grocery store.

Session 1

During the initial interview, Michael expressed reasonable desire to quit smoking and was able to identify a number of reasons why it would be in his best interests to quit. He appreciated the obvious health benefits as well as the aesthetics of being more physically appealing to his girlfriend. Specifically, he realized that his clothes, vehicle, and breath would smell better and Sharon would be inclined to be more physically attentive to him. Michael reported that Sharon would frequently complain about the unappealing smell of his clothes and demanded that he brush his teeth before kissing her. He also was able to identify the cost saving of not smoking without any prompting from David.

Knowing that behavior is maintained even for unhealthy reasons, David asked Michael about the underlying reasons for continuing to smoke. Michael indicated that the brief though effective relaxation response when lighting up and concerns about gaining weight if he did quit smoking were the predominant reasons for continuing to smoke. He also reported that he has some angst about the discomfort he may encounter when he stops smoking and also expressed concern about possible failure with any attempts to quit. When questioned further about this, Michael reported that if he was not able to stop smoking with David's assistance, he was concerned that he may never try to quit smoking in the future knowing his past efforts were futile.

Michael tended to smoke first thing in the morning soon after awakening. He also smoked while driving, provided Sharon was not riding with him. Other smoking times included after meals, during breaks at work, and immediately before going to bed. He reported that he tended to increase his smoking when stressed and under these circumstances was prone to chain-smoking, though this was not frequent. On one occasion he stopped smoking for about five weeks after he had his tonsils removed at age 18. He started smoking again due to the emotional distress experienced after his girlfriend of eight months broke up with him. He immediately began chain-smoking and has not had any extensive nonsmoking periods since that time. He had never smoked "light" cigarettes and did not believe that switching to an alternative brand would be of benefit. He has never used any supplementation to help quit smoking, with the exception of Wellbutrin, as reported above. He tended to smoke alone, though at times there were opportunities for a group of coworkers to take smoke breaks together.

Michael's resultant score of 7 on the Fagerstrom Test for Nicotine Dependence was in the high range for dependence, indicating that he would likely require nicotine supplementation to ease any uncomfortable withdrawal effects once he stopped smoking. His resultant Rotter Scale score of 12 placed him in the borderline range between internal and external locus of control. It was David's sense from talking with Michael that he tended to maintain a reasonable sense of internal control for change, though there were indications that he tended to project blame onto others at times and minimized his own sense of personal accountability.

David provided Michael with the information sheet regarding the changes that occur within the body once a person stops smoking and also asked him to complete the RHETI sampler before returning for his next appointment, which was scheduled one week later.

Session 2

Michael completed the RHETI Sampler and his resultant score was suggestive of a Type Five (Investigator). Within the first few days after his second session, Michael took the RHETI online, which verified results from the Sampler.

Recall that Fives are included within the Thinking Triad and tend to have anxiety about the outer world and concerns about their capacity to cope with it. This data provided a bit more understanding concerning Michael's statement to David during his initial visit about his fear of failure.

Fives are also known for being intense and cerebral. Michael enjoyed working on air and heating units, which of course attracted him to his job as a technician, and during his free time he designed Web pages. Though he was not able to generate adequate income from Web design to support himself, he greatly enjoyed learning how to create images and Web pages and would isolate himself in a spare bedroom during evening hours, at times working through the night, losing track of time and depriving himself of sleep in the process.

Fives are known for being perceptive, innovative, secretive, and isolated, and unfortunately this tended to generate conflict between Michael and Sharon. Though Sharon understood Michael's need for personal space and time, she did not care for the endless hours he would spend in the back bedroom, ignoring her as if she were't even there. Because he did not smoke in their home, Sharon's only contact with him at times was when he would emerge from his study to smoke a cigarette outside.

When functioning well, Fives appreciate the price paid for their social isolation and risk getting in touch with themselves by becoming more grounded in their bodies and their life energy. They become more confident with their abilities to take on leadership roles and manifest the confidence of a healthy Eight. For Michael, his success as a heating and air technician and continued acquisition of knowledge with designing Web pages certainly helped him grow and develop.

Unfortunately, like most Fives, when distressed Michael became scattered and impulsive. He would lose confidence in his ability to work whenever he became unexpectedly challenged at work or when encountering difficulties with learning programming language for Web page designs. This would typically generate conflict in his relationship with Sharon, and with his mother, since these were the predominant significant relationships in his life. It was therefore critical to his treatment to begin to develop interpersonal skills that would foster a greater reliance upon his feelings, as this tends to be the predominant struggle for Fives as well as other personality types in the Thinking Triad.

David reviewed the results of the Enneagram with Michael and asked him to be more cognizant of the times he tended to isolate himself and ignore Sharon. Michael was also encouraged to review some information provided concerning smoking cessation and nicotine withdrawal. Given his relatively elevated Fagerstrom score (7), David encouraged Michael to consider nicotine supplementation in the form of a patch, gum, or lozenge. He provided Michael with information on each of these nicotine alternatives, knowing that, as a Type Five, Michael would need information if he were to come to some decision about how to proceed with his treatment.

Hypnosis was also briefly introduced to Michael and he was given a brochure on hypnotherapy that not only addressed the potential therapeutic benefits, but dispelled many myths associated with this intervention. Michael was rather open to the possibility of hypnosis, so there was no need to overwhelm him with data in an effort to foster compliance. Michael was also assured that there would be other strategies that he could learn that could minimize physical discomfort when he would finally stop smoking and he expressed interest in learning more about them.

Session 3

Michael purchased a 10-week supply of nicotine patches that would gradually be reduced in dosing over time (21 mg, 14 mg, 7 mg). He had not used the patch yet, as he wanted to be a bit more certain about his stop date and have a better sense of support before giving up that last cigarette. He understood the importance of not smoking once he started using the patch and was informed that he should not take the patch off and then smoke a cigarette only to reapply the patch.

During the third session, Michael was introduced to a number of behavioral strategies and interventions to facilitate smoking cessation. He was encouraged to keep his cigarettes in an inconvenient place in his home to foster a greater sense of conscious intention for smoking. He agreed that he could keep them above one of the cabinets in his kitchen and seek the assistance of Sharon to keep them there. Michael also planned to keep his cigarettes in the trunk of his car so that he would have to pull off the road into a safe area to access them. He tended to chain-smoke more frequently in his car than anywhere else and was hoping this would cut down the frequency of smoking at least before he decided to use the patch. David also encouraged Michael to smoke the last cigarette of the evening earlier, thereby prolonging the time between the last cigarette of one day and the first cigarette of the next. Doing so enabled Michael to witness how his body was able to go without smoking a cigarette for up to 10 hours without problem. Michael also agreed that he would begin to smoke his cigarettes with his nondominant left hand and even agreed to hold the cigarette between his middle and ring finger, making it even more uncomfortable and inconvenient. Many people make these positive intentions, though it should be noted that few continue with them if they are not very serious about making more conscious efforts to stop smoking.

Michael was also encouraged to put money in a Mason jar that he would save by not purchasing cigarettes. Like most people he tended to purchase cigarettes by the carton which cost him nearly $50 per week. He would save about $200/month if he became a permanent nonsmoker, not to mention money saved by improving his health and significantly reducing future costs for serious illnesses associated with smoking.

The remainder of the session was dedicated to introducing Michael to hypnosis through some brief trance work. Michael was very eager to initiate hypnosis and informed David that he had done some research of his own on the subject, which of course was no great shock given his Type Five personality. Though he discovered promises of cures for ills that have no known cure, he realized that these exaggerations should not discredit the interventions, only the people attempting to make unreasonable profit from them. He reported that most of what he read seemed very reasonable and certainly "worth a try."

Knowing Michael was concerned about future discomfort, David utilized interventions during the hypnosis session to offer potential relief and comfort. He also employed strategies to help Michael maintain the mindset and identification of himself as a nonsmoker. As can be seen from the transcript below, there were a number of references to how life will be as a nonsmoker. Rather than focusing on what *won't* be there, David emphasized what *will* be present for Michael, the permanent nonsmoker.

After a typical induction utilizing a softer, slower voice that matched Michael's breathing, David employed suggestions to elicit hand, if not arm levitation:

> And as you lay there, your arms by your sides, head on the pillow [descriptive matching], you can continue to feel even more comfortable...your hands may feel *heavy* now...*heavier* than they were when we first started...and with each breath you release, they can feel even *heavier* if you want [This works well in case the person doesn't really want them to feel heavier. Either way, the option is up to the client.]...maybe you can even notice a difference between one hand and the other...one may feel *heavier* than the other, or maybe they have an equal *heaviness* to them, I don't know...just notice how they feel right now...how different they feel there now...one can be *heavier* than the other...maybe you can notice that...maybe your unconscious mind

can notice that...sensing one is *heavier,* the other *lighter...*and one can become *lighter* [this word is said as Michael inhales, matching the rise in his chest with a sense of the hand slightly lifting]...and I'm not sure which one is *lighter* [again stated and timed with an inhalation] or if both perhaps are...*lighter...*as if each breath you take in can make them even *lighter* (at this point, David notices Michael's left hand begin to separate from the chair)...that's right, just like that...as if the gravity around and below that hand became even *lighter...*the weight of the hand, just going away...like it was out in space where there's no gravity to hold it down...feeling like it could just *float* there all on its own...and as it feels *lighter* your unconscious mind can become more available now...available to help you...accessing and mobilizing resources, skills, and abilities (at this point, there is about one inch between Michael's hand and the chair)...it's so *light* that your unconscious mind can allow it to just stay right there...being mindful of how available your unconscious mind is right now to you...knowing that your unconscious mind helps control all of the things that are beyond your conscious control...yet able to help with things like ignoring or *lightening* any sense of discomfort...helping you breathe without having to think about it...beating your heart...helping your body rest while you sleep...keeping you asleep through the night knowing the slightest sounds don't need to awaken you...-moving your body when it needs to move...keeping you healthy...and as your unconscious mind is reminded of all of these things, you can realize how powerful it really is...just like it keeps that hand there feeling so *light,* so comfortable...and as long as it stays light like that your unconscious mind can continue to help you...now and later...now because of how you feel...just notice how *different* you feel right now...and how *different* that is from how you felt when you first came in to my office...that's your unconscious mind helping you...and understanding how it can help you later...just like how an athlete might prepare for an event...imaging how it will go...perceiving and expecting success...and like that you can begin to imagine yourself in your future...how you will *feel different...*how you will do things different...how much better you will feel as Michael the *permanent* nonsmoker...it will be *different...*and *better...*perhaps you can even see how people will respond to you as Michael the permanent nonsmoker...how fresh you and your clothes will smell [note that David does not report how his clothes *won't* smell]...maybe you can even imagine the things that you will be able to do as a healthier and more fit person...and the decisions you will make about how to spend the money that you will now have available to spend...just what would you do with an extra $200 dollars a month or $2400 a year...if it helps you can see how well your unconscious mind can help you see Michael, a permanent nonsmoker, even more vividly...how you can be that person...how the thought of smoking is as foreign to you as it is any other nonsmoker...how even if you get upset or stressed like everybody else, that smoking isn't even a thought...knowing how much healthier you are...how much easier it is to breathe...how you feel *right now* [knowing he most likely felt very good at the moment given his bodily response]...even the thought of lighting up a cigarette makes me feel like I have to cough...how it chokes my breath...how it can choke your breath...and you can imagine anything you like as Michael the permanent nonsmoker...just take some time now while I remain silent for about two minutes of clock time and let your mind be where it is as it settles in and experiences Michael the permanent nonsmoker (two minutes pass and Michael's hand is still slightly elevated)....

Very good...just continue to feel as comfortable as you do [rather nondescript and open-ended] knowing how well your unconscious mind can take this experience in...how it can make it its own...so that it's part of you now...knowing that even if you heard everything I said and remembered everything I said, that's fine...your unconscious mind is wise enough to know what it needs to remember...and even if you consciously don't remember everything, that's okay too...your unconscious mind heard everything it needed to hear and can remember all that it needs to remember to help you now...and later...and when you're ready and you feel that your body has taken in this experience and internalized it, to be there to help you, you can start to become more alert...move or stretch your body and gently open your eyes to get them used to the lighting in the room...it may be brighter in here than you remember...and when you're ready just be more alert...know that as you leave the office today you will take all of the experience that you just had, as it will stay with you to help you now...and later (Michael began to move his right hand then kept it still as his left was still slightly elevated. There was a sense of some resistance to become more alert, so David raised his voice to a little louder level). And you can put your left arm back down as it comes out of trance and as the rest of you becomes more alert...that's right...be more aware of here and now...my voice and my office and the sounds outside of my office (there were some children making some noises in the hallway)...that's right...there you are...so tell me, how did that go for you?

Michael was quiet for a few minutes, staring up at the ceiling, taking a couple of deep breaths, and then he stretched. He told David that he remembered a few things about what happened, but it seemed he was "in another world." He realized that his left hand was elevated but, as he said, "That was okay and I wasn't worried about it." He felt very relaxed and comfortable and, though it had been over an hour since the session started, he reported that for once he didn't have a strong desire to smoke a cigarette like he did the first two times he left David's office. In fact, he planned to see how long he could go without smoking.

He was encouraged to try the suggestions that were recommended at the beginning of the session and to see how long he was able to go without having a really strong desire to smoke again. David encouraged him to not smoke until he had a *really, really* strong desire to do so. He was also encouraged to see how long he could go without smoking between the last cigarette of one day and the first cigarette of the next. If at any time during the week he wanted to start using the patch, he could do so provided he adhered to the instructions and recommendations that accompanied the patch. Of course he was to be sure that he didn't smoke while using the patch if indeed he decided to use it.

Session 4

It had been 10 days between sessions 3 and 4. Michael reported that he hadn't smoked a cigarette until later that evening after last seeing David. He reported that he kept asking himself if he "really, really" needed a cigarette and at 7 PM the answer to the question became a resounding "Yes!" He smoked another at 9 PM and didn't have his next cigarette until 8 AM the following day. He noticed that, as he applied all the behavioral strategies that were discussed during the last session, he didn't feel the need to smoke as frequently. He consciously appreciated how making smoking inconvenient made it less of a necessity than he thought. Two days before this session, he threw away all of his cigarettes and applied the patch, as he was able to go over 12 hours without smoking a cigarette and do so relatively comfortably. He had not smoked a cigarette since starting the patch and, other than a feeling that he described as "itchy," was having no adverse reactions or discomfort. He also started chewing plastic coffee stirs, as he thought this would help curb what he reported to be an "oral fixation".

Session 4 included another hypnosis session that focused on relaxation, on continued perceptions of himself living life as a permanent nonsmoker, and on his body's capacity to heal and soothe any discomfort created by his history of smoking. David also reviewed with Michael the importance of eventually reducing his reliance on the nicotine patch and that physical withdrawal effects from smoking generally persist for only a few days. Utilizing the analogy of suffering through the common cold knowing life will get better helped Michael recognize that the discomfort he may experience is a natural part of healing from the years of abuse that he put his body through by smoking.

Session 5

Michael went through the past week without smoking a cigarette and the day before this session he started a 14-mg patch. Though the manufacturer of the patch recommended using the 21-mg patch for 6 weeks, Michael believed he was ready to reduce the dosage, especially after he and David discussed the expected discomfort that will go away in due time. Though he reported some desire to smoke again, it wasn't particularly strong and, relying again on the question, "Do I *really, really* need a cigarette?" helped him make the conscious effort to not purchase a pack of cigarettes.

During this session, since it appeared that Michael had made reasonable progress, David focused on relapse prevention. Though Michael had had few nonsmoking periods in his life, he was able to appreciate the stressors that may increase his odds of smoking again. Conflicts in his relationship with Sharon were at the top of the list, followed by conflict with his mother and unexpected financial challenges. It was important during this stage of treatment to begin focusing on enhancing Michael's coping skills, which included improving his self-esteem by encouraging more regular exercise, investing in himself by establishing supportive relations, and enhancing financial security by continuing to learn both on and off the job.

Having the personality style of a Type Five challenged matters to some extent, particularly with regard to facilitating a social network. Michael was a rather reserved individual who preferred to keep life simple by keeping people out. Unfortunately, as David pointed out to him, this really wasn't working. In many ways, he had become his own sole source of support and had failed to recognize and benefit from the assistance of others. David encouraged him to take a Web page design course at the local community college, which he eventually did, though with some reluctance. In due time, he actually made some connections with two other men in the class who became close acquaintances (he never referred to them as "friends"). Michael had been walking more than usual, though he had not committed to the idea of exercising regularly, as this has never been part of his persona. Viewing exercise as an investment in himself and his future helped alleviate some anxiety, though he never did join a gym or make exercise a daily ritual in his life even by the time his treatment concluded.

Session 6

It had been two weeks since his last session and Michael reported that he still had not smoked a cigarette. He was chewing coffee stirs "like it was nobody's business," but this was preferred over puffing on a cigarette. Michael reported little desire to actually smoke a cigarette, but still found that he needed to do something to keep his hands busy. He also reported that thus far in his treatment, his greatest struggle was the behavioral aspects of not smoking rather than any discomfort from nicotine withdrawal. He reduced the strength of his nicotine patch to the lowest dosage and indicated that he planned to stay at this dosage for another week or two.

David introduced EFT procedures to Michael, with the understanding that he might still experience some physical discomfort or episodic cravings once he finished with the patch. Though Michael tended to David's instructions as he walked him through the tapping procedures, he balked at the idea of muscle testing. In this particular case, EFT was not something the client expressed an interest in; consequently, this intervention was never addressed again. David did inform Michael that he would be more than willing to review the procedures with him at a later date if he was interested in learning how to reduce cravings in particular.

With only 15 minutes to go in the session, Michael requested a brief hypnosis session. Here is a partial transcript from that session:

> [J]ust make yourself as comfortable as you can be, Michael…taking in a slow deep breath, holding for a moment and gently releasing as you get ready to *go into trance*…that's right, and you can do that one or two or more times…to help *go into trance*…to help you take this opportunity to settle your conscious mind…to give it that time out it needs…to *go into trance*…and allow your unconscious mind to be more available…to help you now and later…you know there are so many ways to *go into trance*…we all *go into trance* many times each day…driving in the car and getting lost in thought… arriving at our destination sooner than expected…not recalling passing a certain landmark…getting lost in a movie to such an extent that you start talking to the television or movie screen…knowing no one can really hear you…but just talking automatically…without conscious thought…or maybe for you getting lost in your work…getting lost in your Web design and losing track of time…just like that you can *go into trance*…over time, you will learn to find you own way *into trance*, finding ways to even go in *deeper* if you want…feel the comfort, the soothing, and healing abilities of each breath that you take in…just imagine how each breath of *fresh air* [as opposed to cigarette smoke] allows you to relax more comfortably…and how each breath allows you to *relax* and feel more comfortable for longer periods of time [unlike cigarettes, which provide a sense of relaxation for no more than a few minutes]…notice right now how you feel [there is ample evidence from his slowed breathing rate and relaxed facial muscles that he is very comfortable]…imagine how this feeling can stay with you…helping you *go into trance*…*deeper* if you want…you can really decide…it's up to you…you have the controls, the volume button to turn it all up and give yourself that *even deeper* sense of comfort…or stay right where you are *in trance*…or if

you need you can even lighten your *trance* and not go in any *deeper* [using interspersal, recommending a deeper trance to the subconscious mind while permitting the conscious mind to make its own decision]...for some people, just a light *trance* is helpful...there is no need to *go deeper* or feel *more comfortable* than they already feel...either way, you can make this trance a trance that works for you...just continue to think whatever you think, feel whatever you feel...notice how *different* you feel now...is this more comfortable...healthier for you...feeling this way perhaps helps you feel how you can manage stress in your day...how your unconscious mind can help you access these feelings, these resources...helping you manage...adapting to stress as a nonsmoker...maybe right now you have an idea of how much time has passed since we started this session...how long does it seem...and isn't it interesting how time can *feel* different even though every minute is the same...60 seconds is 60 seconds...but sometimes time can move faster, like when you sleep...or when you get distracted by something that grabs your attention...how your body can feel uncomfortable one minute but better the next and you didn't even know it...when do you really appreciate that a cold or headache is gone...don't you notice it well after it's over...not at that very minute...and like that, your subconscious mind can allow your body to be distracted...to not be so aware of every discomfort...like the time I knew I had to go to the bathroom before the movie started...but I didn't want to leave the theatre and risk missing the beginning so I sat there and waited for the movie to start...and it wasn't until it was over that I remembered I still had to go to the bathroom...that was my unconscious mind...putting that discomfort out of mind...keeping it away so I could feel comfortable...like you feel comfortable right now...

This session concluded, like the prior session, with David requesting Michael to be more consciously aware of his surroundings. As he stretched and prepared himself to leave the office, Michael informed David that he really got in touch with his breathing. Imaging it being healthier provided him with energy and relaxation at the same time. Though David never specifically stated this during the session, it was something that Michael experienced. When clients report such experiences, it is usually confirmation that the hypnosis was helpful, as the unconscious mind is accessing and mobilizing resources that previously had not been used to their fullest potential.

Session 7

One week after his last session, Michael reported that he was still not smoking and gaining greater confidence that he would never smoke again. He had been relying less on his coffee stirs, though he had substituted nicotine gum for the patch. He had been chewing about six pieces of gum each day and finding this seemed helpful at keeping any unwanted side effects from nicotine withdrawal at bay. He did find the flavor a bit unappealing and also experienced some "chalky buildup" at the corners of his mouth. David encouraged him to keep his pieces of gum limited to about six, as any more may increase the nicotine in his blood stream and ultimately defeat the purpose of reducing nicotine consumption.

He had few if any significant stressors to challenge his coping skills, but he indicated that even if life did become difficult he didn't think that he would consider smoking as an option. His girlfriend was thrilled that he was not smoking and frequently praised him for his efforts and success. Like David, Sharon cautioned Michael about his use of nicotine gum and encouraged him to drop one piece of gum every other day, so that within 2 weeks he wouldn't be using any nicotine supplementation at all. He told David he thought this a reasonable plan, but, knowing himself, he was just as likely to quit the gum cold turkey.

Though offered the opportunity for hypnosis during this session, Michael declined, stating that he didn't think it was necessary. He was feeling very confident about not smoking and thought it was only a matter of time before he quit using nicotine gum and, in his words, was "well on my way to being a permanent nonsmoker." He made an appointment for 2 weeks later, at which time he hoped he would cease all nicotine supplementation.

Session 8

As desired, Michael stopped chewing the nicotine gum without adverse impact. He had gone 3 days prior to this session without smoking or using any supplement whatsoever. There had been a number of stressful events between visits, including a threat of job loss that fortunately did not come to fruition. Because of the downturn in the economy, new home sales had steadily declined. The owner of his company informed all technicians that he may need to lay them off and at the very least may have to discontinue their health care plan to cut costs in an effort to preserve jobs. Though two other technicians lost their jobs, Michael did not. Though he was concerned about the very real possibility of losing his job, he had no desire to smoke cigarettes again. Since smoking his last cigarette, Michael saved $350 and planned to put this money toward his honeymoon.

His cravings were limited and when they occurred he usually found ways to distract himself, including taking a walk or reading a book. He acknowledged that many cravings occurred while driving his car, and that he continued to keep some plastic coffee stirs in the glove box to help satiate any desire to smoke. Interestingly, he found second-hand cigarette smoke irritating and preferred nonsmoking establishments to those with smoking sections.

During this session, David asked Michael to identify all of the benefits he had experienced to date since he stopped smoking. In addition to the money savings reported above, Michael indicated that his relationship with his fiancé had become more intimate (since he didn't smell like an ashtray), his health and energy levels had improved, and he felt more confident about himself since he was able to modify his habits and become a permanent nonsmoker.

Michael followed up with David 6 weeks later and had still not smoked a cigarette. He had saved over $400 and was looking forward to saving more money by not smoking. He happened to find an old pack of cigarettes that he had hidden, "in case of an emergency" and had no qualms about throwing it away. This was Michael's last visit with David and there has been no follow-up with him as of the writing of this text.

CONCLUSION

The case studies included in this chapter were provided for the general purpose of illustrating in more pragmatic terms the comprehensive treatment plan and interventions offered for helping people change unwanted behavior. Each case study begins with information gathered from the personal history interview, and includes personality dynamics generated from the Enneagram, interventions based in part on results from the Enneagram, transcriptions from hypnosis sessions, and for one case applications of Energy Psychology. The hypnosis transcripts for both cases offer examples of specific techniques, including utilization, linking, and descriptive matching. We hope we provided you with ample information to use for your own work with habit control. We also hope that you gained an understanding of the importance and necessity of individualizing treatment tailored on impressions from the clinical interview, personal history, results of the Enneagram, and impressions that continue to be generated as treatment unfolds. Maintaining a sense of flexibility is crucial to offering effective treatment, though it should be apparent from the subject matter discussed in each chapter that we clearly recommend specific strategies for the treatment of unwanted habits.

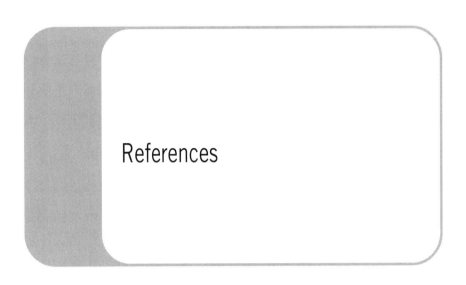

References

Abraham, S., & Llewellyn-Jones, D. (2001). *Eating disorders: The facts.* New York: Oxford University Press.

American Psychiatric Association. (2000). *Diagnostic and statistical manual of mental disorders* (4ᵗʰ ed., text rev.). Washington, DC: American Psychiatric Press.

American Psychological Association, Division of Psychological Hypnosis. (1993). Hypnosis. *Psychological Hypnosis,* pp. 2–3.

Andersen, M. R., Leroux, B. G., Bricker, J. B., Rajan, K. B., & Peterson, A.V . (2004). Antismoking parenting practices are associated with reduced rates of adolescent smoking. *Archives of Pediatric and Adolescent Medicine, 158*(4), 348–352.

Anderssen, N., & Wold, B. (1992). Parental and peer influences on leisure-time physical activity in young adolescents. *Research Quarterly for Exercise and Sport, 63,* 341–348.

Andrade, A. M., Greene, G. W., & Melanson, K. J. (2008). Eating slowly led to decreases in energy intake within meals in healthy women. *Journal of the American Dietetic Association, 108*(7), 1186–1191.

Arterburn, D. E., Maciejewski, M. L., & Tsevat, J. (2005). Impact of morbid obesity on medical expenditures in adults. *International Journal of Obesity, 29*(3), 334–339.

Bader, D. M. (2002). *Zen Judaism: For you a little enlightenment.* New York: Harmony Books.

Bandler, R., & Grinder, J. (1975). *Patterns of the hypnotic techniques of Milton Erickson, M.D. Volume 1.* Cupertino, CA: Meta.

Beyer, K., & Teuber, S. S. (2005). Food allergy diagnostics: Scientific and unproven procedures. *Current Opinion in Allergy and Clinical Immunology, 5*(3), 261–266.

Bliss, E. L. (1986). *Multiple personality, allied disorders, and hypnosis.* New York: Oxford University Press.

Bolocofsky, D. N., Spinler, D., & Coulthard-Morris, L. (1985). Effectiveness of hypnosis as an adjunct to behavioral weight management. *Journal of Clinical Psychology, 41*(1), 35–41.

Bridge, J. A., Iyengar, S., Salary, C. B., Barbe, R. P., Birmaher, B., Pincus, H. A., et al. (2007). Clinical response and risk for reported suicidal ideation and suicide attempts in pediatric antidepressant treatment: a meta-analysis of randomized controlled studies. *Journal of the American Medical Association, 297*(15), 1683–1696.

Cairella, G., Ciarall, F., Longo, P., Rebella, V, Molino, N, D'Urso, A., et al. (2007). Smoking cessation and weight gain. *Annali di igiene: Medicina preventiva e di comunità, 19*(1), 73–81.

Callahan, R. J. (1990). *How executives overcome the fear of public speaking and other phobias.* New York: McGraw-Hill.

Callan, D. E., Tsytsarev, V., Hanakawa, T., Callan, A. M., Katsuhara, M., Fukuyama, H., et al. (2006). Song and speech: Brain regions involved with perception and covert production. *Neruoimage, 31*(3), 1327–1242.

Carmody, T. P., Duncan, C., Simon, J. A., Solkowitz, S., Huggins, J., Lee, S., et al. (2008). Hypnosis for smoking cessation: A randomized trial. *Nicotine and Tobacco Research, 10*(5), 811–818.

Centers for Disease Control and Prevention. (2002). Annual smoking-attributable mortality, years of potential life lost, and economic costs—U.S., 1995–1999. *Morbidity and Mortality Weekly Reports, 55*(14), 300–303.

Centers for Disease Control and Prevention. (2006). State-specific prevalence of obesity among adults—United States, 2005. *Morbidity and Mortality Weekly Reports, 55*(36), 985–988.

Chassin, L., Presson, C., Rose, J., Sherman, S. J., & Prost, J. (2002). Parental smoking cessation and adolescent smoking. *Journal of Pediatric Psychology, 27*(6), 485–496.

Covey, S. R. (1989). *The 7 habits of highly effective people.* New York: Free Press.

Cramer, S. C., Orr, E. L., Cohen, M. J., & Lacourse, M. G. (2007). Effects of motor imagery training after chronic, complete spinal cord injury. *Experimental Brain Research, 177*(2), 233–242.

Dannenberg, A., Burton, D., & Jackson, R. (2004). Economic and environmental costs of obesity: The impact on airlines. *American Journal of Preventive Medicine, 27*(3), 264.

Davis, B., & Carpenter, C. (2009). Proximity of fast-food restaurants to schools and adolescent obesity. *American Journal of Public Health, 99*(3), 505-510

Debus, A. G., & Multhauf, R. P. (1966). *Alchemy and chemistry in the seventheenth century.* Los Angeles: William Andres Clark Memorial Library, University of California.

Delazer, M., Domahs, F., Bartha, L., Brenneis, C., Lochy, A., Trieb, T., et al. (2003). Learning complex arithmetic—an fMRI study. *Brain Research. Cognitive Brain Research, 18*(1), 76–88.

de Lorgeril, M., Salen, P., Martin, J., Monjaud, I., Delay, J., & Mamelle, N. (1999). Mediterranean diet, traditional risk factors, and the rate of cardiovascular complications after myocardial infarction. *Circulation, 99*, 779–785.

Doggrell, S. A. (2007). Which is the best primary medication for long-term smoking cessation-nicotine replacement therapy, bupropion, or varenicline? *Expert Opinion on Pharmacotherapy, 8*(17), 2903–2915.

Dolan, S. L., Sacco, K. A., Termine, A., Seyal, A. A., Dudas, M. M., Yessicchio, J. C., et al. (2004). Neuropsychological deficits are associated with smoking cessation treatment failure in patients with schizophrenia. *Schizophrenia Research, 70*(2–3), 263–275.

Dolezal, B. A., & Potteiger, J. A. (1998). Concurrent resistance and endurance training influence basal metabolic rate in nondieting individuals. *Journal of Applied Physiology, 85*(2), 695–700.

Drewnowski, A., Krahn, D. D., Demitrack, M. A., Nairn, K., & Gosnell, B. A. (1992). Taste responses and preferences for sweet high-fat foods: Evidence for opioid involvement. *Physiology and Behavior, 51*(2), 371–379.

Dyer, D. D. (2004). *The power of intention.* Carlsbad: Hay House.

Elkins, G., Marcus, J., Bates, J., Hasan Rajab, M., & Cook, T. (2006). Intensive hypnotherapy for smoking cessation: A prospective study. *International Journal of Clinical and Experimental Hypnosis, 54*(3), 303–315.

Elkins, G. R., & Rajab, M. H. (2004). Clinical hypnosis for smoking cessation: Preliminary results of a three-session intervention. *International Journal of Clinical and Experimental Hypnosis, 52*(1), 73–81.

Erickson, M. (1966). The interspersal hypnotic technique for symptom correction and pain control. *American Journal of Clinical Hypnosis, 8,* 83–88.

Erickson, M. (1983). *Healing in hypnosis: The seminars, workshops, and lectures of Milton H. Erickson* (Vol. 1). New York: Irvington.

Erickson, M. (1985). *Life reframing in hypnosis: The seminars, workshops, and lectures of Milton H. Erickson* (Vol. II). New York: Irvington.

Erickson, M., & Rossi, E. (1979). *Hypnotherapy: An exploratory casebook.* New York: Irvington.

Erickson, M., Rossi, E., & Rossi, S. (1976). *Hypnotic realities: The induction of clinical hypnosis and forms of indirect suggestion.* New York: Irvington.

Feinstein, D., & Eden, D. (2008). Six pillars of energy medicine: Clinical strengths of a complimentary paradigm. *Alternative Therapies in Health and Medicine, 14*(1), 44–54.

Filozof, C., Fernandez Pinilla, M. C., & Fernandez-Cruz, A. (2004). Smoking cessation and weight gain. *Obesity Reviews, 5*(2), 95–103.

Flood, J. E., Roe, L. S., & Rolls, B. J. (2006). The effect of increased beverage portion size on energy intake at a meal. *Journal of the American Dietetic Association, 106*(12), 1984–1990.

Flood-Obbagy, J. E., & Rolls, B. J. (2008). The effect of fruit in different forms on energy intake and satiety at a meal. *Appetite, 52*(2), 416-422.

Foster-Powell, K., Holt, S. H. A., & Brand-Miller, J. C. (2002). International table of glycemic index and glycemic load values: 2002. *American Journal of Clinical Nutrition, 76*(1), 5-56.

Freud, S. (1949). *An outline of psycho-analysis.* New York: W.W. Norton.

Furman, M. E., & Gallo, F. P. (2000). *The neurophysics of human behavior.* Boca Raton: CRC Press.

Gallo, F. P. (2005). *Energy psychology: explorations at the interface of energy, cognition, behavior, and health* (2nd ed.). Boca Raton: CRC Press.

Gallwey, W. T. (1973). *The inner game of tennis.* New York: Random House.

Gallwey, W. T. (1981). *The inner game of golf.* New York: Random House

Gallwey, W. T. (2000). *The inner game of work: Focus, learning, pleasure, and mobility in the workplace.* New York: Random House.

Garakani, A., Mathew, S. J., & Charney, D. S. (2006). Neurobiology of anxiety disorders and implications for treatment. *Mount Sinai Journal of Medicine, 73*(7), 941–949.

Garrison, F. H. (1966). *History of medicine.* Philadelphia: W.B. Saunders.

Garrow, J. S., & Webster, J. (1985). Quetelet's index (W/H2) as a measure of fatness. *International Journal of Obesity, 9,* 147–153.

George, T. P., Termine, A., Sacco, K. A., Allen, T. M., Reutenauer, E., Vessicchio, J. C., et al. (2006). A preliminary study of the effects of cigarette smoking on prepulse inhibition in schizophrenia: Involvement of nicotinic receptor mechanisms. *Schizophrenia Research, 87*(1–3), 307–315.

Glenville, M. (2001). *The natural health handbook for women.* London: Piatkus Publishers.

Gluck, M. E., Geliebter, A., & Satov, T. (2001). Night eating syndrome is associated with depression, low self-esteem, reduced daytime hunger, and less weight loss in obese outpatients. *Obesity Research, 9*(4), 264–267.

Grimal, N. (1988). *A history of ancient Egypt.* Boston: Blackwell Publishing.

Grogan, S., Fry, G., Gough, B., & Conner, M. (2009). Smoking to stay thin or giving up to save face? Young men and women talk about appearance concerns and smoking. *British Journal of Health Psychology, 14*(1), 175–186.

Gunji, A., Ishii, R., Chau, W., Kakigi, R., & Pantev, C. (2007). Rhythmic brain activities related to singing in humans. *Neuroimage, 34*(1), 426–434.

Gutschall, M. D., Miller, C. K., Mitchell, D. C., & Lawrence, F. R. (2009). A randomized behavioral trial targeting glycaemic index improves dietary, weight, metabolic outcomes in patients with type 2 diabetes. *Public Health Nutrition, 23*(1), 1–9.

Hall, S., Lewith, G., Brien, S., & Little, P. (2008). A review of the literature in applied and specialised kinesiology. *Forschende Komplementarmedizin, 15*(1), 40–46.

Heatherton, T. F., Kozlowski, L. T., Frecker, R. C., & Fagerstrom, K. O. (1991). The Fagerstrom Test for Nicotine Dependence: A revision of the Fagerstrom Tolerance Questionnaire. *British Journal of Addiction, 86*(9), 1119–1127.

Hull, C. L. (1962). Psychology of the scientist: IV. Passages from the "idea books" of Clark L. Hull. *Perceptual and Motor Skills, 15,* 807–882.

International Association of Pure Hypnoanalysts. (2007). *History of hypnosis.* Retrieved October 6, 2009, from www.successfulhypnotherapy.com/hypnosishtml.

International Diabetes Federation. (2004). Diabetes and obesity: Time to act. *Diabetes Care, 27,* 2067–2073.

Ischebeck, A., Zamarian, L., Schocke, M., & Delazer, M. (2009). Flexible transfer of knowledge in mental arithmetic—An fMRI study. *Neuroimage, 44*(3), 1103–1112.

Jackson, K. A., Byrne, N. M., Magarey, A. M., & Hills, A. P. (2008). Minimizing random error in dietary intakes assessed by 24-h recall in overweight and obese adults. *European Journal of Clinical Nutrition, 62*(4), 537–543.

Johnson, D. L. (1997). Weight loss for women: Studies of smokers and non-smokers using hypnosis and multicomponent treatments with and without overt aversion. *Psychological Reports, 80*(3), 931–933.

Kawachi, I., Troisi, R. J., Rotnitzky, A. G., Coakley, E. H., & Colditz, G. A. (1996). Can physical activity minimize weight gain in women after smoking cessation? *American Journal of Public Health, 86*(7), 999–1004.

Knauer, S. (2002). *Recovering from sexual abuse, addictions, and compulsive behaviors: "Numb" survivors.* New York: Haworth Press.

Kodl, M. M., Willenbring, M. L., Gravely, A., Nelson, D. B., & Joseph, A. M. (2008). The impact of depressive symptoms on alcohol and cigarette consumption following treatment for alcohol and nicotine dependence. *Alcoholism, Clinical and Experimental Research, 32*(1), 92–99.

Lancelot, M. (2007). *Gripped by gambling.* Tuscon, AZ: Wheatmark.

Lawson, A., & Calderon, L. (1997). Interexaminer agreement for applied kinesiology manual muscle testing. *Perceptual and Motor Skills, 84*(2), 539–546.

Lehner, M. (1997). *The complete pyramids: Solving the ancient mysteries.* London: Thames & Hudson.

Lemmer, J. T., Ivey, F. M., Ryan, A. S., Martel, G. F., Hurlbut, D. E., Metter, J. E., et al. (2001). Effect of strength training on resting metabolic rate and physical activity: Age and gender comparisons. *Medicine and Science in Sports Medicine, 33*(4), 532–541.

Lois, N., Abdelkader, E., Reglitz, K., Garden, C., & Ayres, J. G. (2008). Environmental tobacco smoke exposure and eye disease. *British Journal of Ophthalmology, 92*(10), 1304–1310.

Lynne, S., & Rhue, J. (Eds.). (1991). *Theories of hypnosis: Current models and perspectives.* New York: Guilford.

Medical News Today. (2004). *Youngest type II diabetes child ever is five-years-old.* Retrieved May 9, 2004, from www.medicalnewstoday.com/?articles/?8111.php.

Mei, Z., Grummer-Strawn, L. M., Pietrobelli, A., Goulding, A., Goran, M. I., & Dietz, W. H. (2002). Validity of body mass index compared with other body-composition screening indexes for the assessment of body fatness in children and adolescents. *American Journal of Clinical Nutrition, 75*(6), 978–985.

Mehta, H., Nazzal, K., & Sadikot, R. T. (2008). Cigarette smoking and innate immunity. *Inflammation Resource, 57*(11), 497–503.

Meyers, L. (2007). Serenity now: East meets west as psychologists embrace ancient traditions to enhance modern practice. *Monitor on Psychology, 38*(11), 32–34.

Mikkonen, P., Leino-Arjas, P., Remes, J., Zitting, P., Taimela, S., & Karppinen, J. (2008). Is smoking a risk factor for low back pain in adolescents? A prospective cohort study. *Spine, 33*(5), 527–532.

Miller, C. K., Gutschall, M. D., & Mitchell, D. C. (2009). Change in food choices following a glycemic load intervention in adults with type 2 diabetes. *Journal of the American Diabetic Association, 109*(2), 319–324.

Miller, J. B., Foster-Powell, K., & Atkinson, F. (2007). *The new glucose revolution shopper's guide to GI values 2008: The authoritative source of glycemic index value for more than 1000 foods.* New York: De Capo Press.

Miller, J. B., Foster-Powell, K., & McMillan-Price, J. (2005). *The low GI diet cookbook: 100 simple, delicious smart-carb recipes—The proven way to lose weight and eat for lifelong health (glucose revolution).* New York: De Capo Press.

Miller, J. B., Foster-Powell, K., & Sandall, P. (2005). *The new glucose revolution: Low GI eating made easy.* New York: Marlow.

Mizoue, T., Ueda, R., Tokui, N., Hino, Y., & Yoshimura, T. (1998). Body mass decrease after initial gain following smoking cessation. *International Journal of Epidemiology, 27*(6), 984–988.

Morita, A. (2007). Tobacco smoke causes premature skin aging. *Journal of Dermatological Science, 48*(3), 169–175.

Muller, K., Butefisch, C. M., & Seitz, R. J. (2007). Mental practice improves hand function after hemiparetic stroke. *Restorative Neurology and Neuroscience, 25*(5–6), 501–511.

National Institutes of Health. (2006). National Institutes of Health State-of-the-Science Conference statement: Tobacco use: Prevention, cessation, and control. *Annals of Internal Medicine, 145,* 839–844.

National Institutes of Health: National Heart, Lung, and Blood Institute. (1998). Clinical guidelines on the identification, evaluation, and treatment of overweight and obesity in adults. *NIH Publication No. 98-4083.*

Novotny, J. A., Rumpler, W. V., Riddick, H., Hebert, J. R., Rhodes, D., Judd, J. T., et al. (2003). Personality characteristics as predictors of underreporting of energy intake on 24-hour dietary recall interviews. *Journal of the American Dietetic Association, 103*(9), 1146–1151.

Ogden, C. L., Carroll, M. D., Curtin, L. R., McDowell, M. A., Tabak, C. J., & Flegal, K. M. (2006). Prevalence of overweight and obesity in the United States, 1999–2004. *Journal of the American Medical Association, 295*(13), 1549–1555.

O'Hanlon, B. (2007, December). *Metaphors be with you: How to use stories and rituals as powerful tools in changework.* Seminar presented at the National Institute for the Clinical Application of Behavioral Medicine, Hilton Head, SC.

O'Hanlon, W. H. (1987). *Taproots: Underlying principles of Milton Erickson's therapy and hypnosis.* New York: W.W. Norton.

O'Hanlon, W. H., & Martin, M. (1992). *Solution oriented hypnosis: An Ericksonian approach.* New York: W. W. Norton.

Olsson, C. J., Jonsson, B., & Nyberg, L. (2008). Internal imagery training in active high jumpers. *Scandinavian Journal of Psychology, 49*(2), 133–140.

Osler, W. (2004). *The evolution of modern medicine.* Whitefish, MT: Kessinger Publishing.

Ozdemir, E., Norton, A., & Schlaug, G. (2006). Shared and distinct neural correlates of singing and speaking. *Neuroimage, 33*(2), 628–635.

Palmer, K. T., Syddall, H., Cooper, C., & Coggon, D. (2003). Smoking and musculoskeletal disorders: Findings from a British national survey. *Annals of the Rheumatic Diseases, 62*(1), 33–36.

Parsons, A. C., Shraim, M., Inglis, J., Aveyard, P., & Hajek, P. (2009). Interventions for preventing weight gain after smoking cessation. *Cochrane Database of Systematic Reviews, 21*(1), CD006219.

Pereira, M. A., Kartashov, A. I., Ebbeling, C. B., Van Horn, L., Slattery, M. L., Jacobs, D. R., et al. (2005). Fast-food habits, weight gain, and insulin resistance (the CARDIA study): 15-year prospective analysis. *Lancet, 365*(9453), 4–5.

Perkins, K. A. (1992). Effects of tobacco smoking on caloric intake. *British Journal of Addiction, 87*(2), 193–205.

Perkins, K. A. (1993). Weight gain following smoking cessation. *Journal of Consulting and Clinical Psychology, 61*(5), 768–777.

Poehlman, E. T., Denino, W. F., Beckett, T., Kinaman, K. A., Dionne, I. J., Dvorak, R., et al. (2002). Effects of endurance and resistance training on total daily energy expenditure in young women: A controlled randomized trial. *Journal of Clinical Endocrinology and Metabolism, 87*(3), 1004–1009.

Powell, K., & Powell, A. (2007). *Top 10 New Year's resolutions.* Retrieved January 1, 2007, from http:/?/?pittsburgh.about.com/?od/?holidays/?tp/?resolutions.?htm

Pratley, R., Nicklas, B., Rubin, M., Miller, J., Smith, A., Smith, M., et al. (1994). Strength training increases resting metabolic rate and norepinephrine levels in healthy 50- to 65-yr-old men. *Journal of Applied Psychology, 76*(1), 133–137.

Prochaska, J. O., & DiClemente, C. C. (1992). Stages of change in the modification of problem behaviors. *Progressive Behavior Modification, 8,* 183–218.

Rachlin, H. (1990). Why do people gamble and keep gambling despite heavy losses? *Psychological Science, 1,* 294–297.

Ragland, D. R., & Brand, R. J. (1988). Coronary heart disease mortality in the Western Collaborative Group Study. Follow-up experience of 22 years. *American Journal of Epidemiology, 127*(3), 462–475.

Riso, D. R., & Hudson, R. (1999). *The wisdom of the Enneagram: The complete guide to psychological and spiritual growth for the nine personality types.* New York: Bantam Books.

Riso, D. R., & Hudson, R. (2003). *Discovering your personality type: The essential introduction to the Enneagram, revised and expanded.* New York: Houghton Mifflin.

Rolls, B. J. (2005). *The Volumetrics Eating Plan: Techniques and recipes for feeling full on fewer calories.* New York: HarperCollins.

Rolls, B. J., Roe, L. S., & Meengs, J. S. (2006). Reductions in portion size and energy density of foods are additive and lead to sustained decreases in energy intake. *American Journal of Clinical Nutrition, 83*(1), 11–17.

Rolls, B. J., Roe, L. S., & Meengs, J. S. (2006). Larger portion sizes lead to a sustained increase in energy intake over two days. *Journal of the American Dietetic Association, 106*(4), 543–549.

Rosen, S. (1982). *My voice will go with you: The teaching tales of Milton H. Erickson, M.D.* New York: W. W. Norton.

Rosenman, R. H., Brand, R. J., Jenkins, D., Friedman, M., Straus, R., & Wurm, H. (1975). Coronary heart disease in Western Collaborative Group Study. Final follow-up experience of 8 1/2 years. *Journal of the American Medical Association, 233*(8), 872–877.

Rotter, J. B. (1966). Generalized expectancies of internal versus external control of reinforcements. *Psychological Monographs, 80* (Whole no. 609).

Rowe, J. E. (2005). The effects of EFT on long-term psychological symptoms. *Counseling and Clinical Psychology, 2*(3), 104–111.

Saules, K. K., Pomerleau, C. S., Snedecor, S. M., Brouwer, R. N., & Rosenberg, E. E. (2004). Effects of disordered eating and obesity on weight, craving, and food intake during ad libitum smoking and abstinence. *Eating Behaviors, 5*(4), 353–363.

Schmitt, W. H., & Leisman, G. (1998). Correlation of applied kinesiology muscle testing findings with serum immunoglobulin levels for food allergies. *International Journal of Neuroscience, 96*(3–4), 237–244.

Silagy, C., Lancaster, T., Stead, L., Mant, D., & Fowler, G. (2002). Nicotine replacement therapy for smoking cessation. *Cochrane Database of Systematic Reviews, 4,* CD000146.

Silbernagel, M. S., Short, S. E., & Ross-Stewart, L. C. (2007). Athletes' use of exercise imagery during weight training. *Journal of Strength and Conditioning Research, 21*(4), 1077–1081.

Simopoulos, A. P. (2006). Evolutionary aspects of diet, the omega-6/omega-3 ration and genetic variation: Nutritional implications for chronic diseases. *Biomedicine & Pharmacotherapy, 60*(9), 502–507.

Simopoulos, A. P. (2002). Omega-3 fatty acids in inflammation and autoimmune diseases. *Journal of the American College of Nutrition, 21*(6), 495–505.

Speakman, J. R., & Selman, C. (2003). Physical activity and resting metabolic rate. *Proceedings of the Nutrition Society, 62*(3), 621–634.

Speechly, D. P., Rogers, G. G., & Buffenstein, R. (1999). Acute appetite reduction associated with an increased frequency of eating in obese males. *International Journal of Obesity and Related Metabolic Disorders, 23*(11), 1151–1159.

Stayner, L., Bena, J., Sasco, A. J., Smith, R., Steenland, K., Kreuzer, M., et al. (2007). Lung cancer risk and workplace exposure to environmental tobacco smoke. *American Journal of Public Health, 97*(3), 545–551.

Strine, T. W., Okoro, C. A., Chapman, D. P., Balluz, L. S., Ford, E. S., Ajani, U. A., et al. (2005). Health-related quality of life and health risk behaviors among smokers. *American Journal of Preventive Medicine, 28*(2), 182–187.

Stucky-Ropp, R. C., & DiLorenzo, T. M. (1993). Determinants of exercise in children. *Preventive Medicine, 22,* 880–889.

Substance Abuse & Mental Health Services Administration. (2006). *Results from the 2005 National Survey on Drug Use and Health: National findings* (NSDUH Series H-30, DHHS Publication No. SMA 06-4194). Rockville, MD: SAMHSA Office of Applied Studies.

Sullivan, E. L., Daniels, A. J., Koegler, F. H., & Cameron, J. L. (2005). Evidence in female rhesus monkeys (*Macaca mulatta*) that nighttime caloric intake is not associated with weight gain. *Obesity Research, 13*(12), 2072–2080.

Sullivan, E. L., Koegler, F. H., & Cameron, J. L. (2006). Individual differences in physical activity are closely associated with changes in body weight in adult female rhesus monkeys (*Macaca mulatta*). *American Journal of Physiology, Regulatory, Integrative, and Comparative Physiology, 291*(3), 633–642.

Tostes, R. C., Carneiro, F. S., Lee, A. J., Giachini, F. R., Leite, R., Osawa, Y., et al. (2008). Cigarette smoking and erectile dysfunction: Focus on NO bioavailability and ROS generation. *Journal of Sex Medicine, 5*(6), 1284–1295.

Trost, S. G., Sallis, J. F., Pate, R. R., Freedson, P. S., Taylor, W. C., & Dowda, M. (2003). Evaluating a model of parental influence on youth physical activity. *American Journal of Preventive Medicine, 24*(4), 277–282.

U.S. Department of Health and Human Services. (1990). The health benefits of smoking cessation. Rockville, MD: U.S. Department of Health and Human Services, Public

Health Service, Centers for Disease Control, Center for Chronic Disease Prevention and Health Promotion, Office on Smoking and Health.

U.S. Department of Health and Human Services. (2004). *The Health Consequences of Smoking: A Report of the Surgeon General.* U.S. Department of Health and Human Services, Centers for Disease Control and Prevention, National Center for Chronic Disease Prevention and Health Promotion, Office on Smoking and Health.

U.S. Department of Health and Human Services, Centers for Disease Control and Prevention. (2006). *The health consequences of involuntary exposure to tobacco smoke: A report of the Surgeon General* (Office of the Surgeon General). Rockville, MD: U.S. Department of Health and Human Services.

Van Etten, L. M., Westerterp, K. R., Verstappen, F. T., Boon, B. J., & Saris, W. H. (1997). Effect of an 18-wk weight-training program on energy expenditure and physical activity. *Journal of Applied Physiology, 82*(1), 298–304.

Vinci, P., Serrao, M., Pierelli, F., Sandrini, G., & Santilli, V. (2006). Lower limb manual muscle testing in the early stages of Charcot-Marie Tooth disease type 1A. *Functional Neurology, 21*(3), 159–163.

Waite, T. R. (2007). *Plugged in: A clinicians' and families' guide to online video game addiction.* Frederick, MD: PublishAmerica.

Wajchenberg, B. L. (2000). Subcutaneous and visceral adipose tissue: Their relation to the metabolic syndrome. *Endocrine Review 21*(6), 697–738.

Walker, M. B. (1989). Some problems with the concept of "gambling addiction": Should theories of addiction be generalized to include excessive gambling? *Journal of Gambling Behavior, 5,* 179–200.

Wang, Z., Heshka, S., Zhang, K., Boozer, C. N., & Heymsfield, S. B. (2001). Resting energy expenditure: systematic organization and critique of prediction methods. *Obesity Research, 9*(5), 331–336.

Wansink, B. (2004). Environmental factors that increase the food intake and consumption volume of unknowing consumers. *Annual Review of Nutrition, 24,* 455–479.

Wansink, B., & Chandon, P. (2006). Can low-fat nutrition labels lead to obesity? *Journal of Marketing Research, 43*(4), 605–617.

Wansink, B., & Cheney, M. M. (2005). Super bowls: Serving bowl size and food consumption. *Journal of the American Medical Association, 293*(14), 1727–1728.

Wansink, B., Painter, J. E., & Lee, Y. K. (2006). The office candy dish: Proximity's influence on estimated and actual consumption. *International Journal of Obesity, 30*(5), 871–875.

Wansink, B., Painter, J. E., & North, J. (2005). Bottomless bowls: Why visual cues of portion size may influence intake. *Obesity Research, 13*(1), 93–100.

Wansink, B., Payne, C. R., & Chandon, P. (2007). Internal and external cues of meal cessation: The French paradox redux? *Obesity, 15*(2), 2920–2924.

Watters, S. O. (2001). *Real solutions for overcoming internet addictions.* Kent, CT: Vine Books.

Webster's new world dictionary: Second college edition. (1982). New York: Simon & Schuster.

Wilkinson, A. V., Shete, S., & Prokhorov, A. V. (2008). The moderating role of parental smoking on their children's attitudes toward smoking among a predominantly minority sample: A cross-sectional analysis. *Substance Abuse, Treatment, Prevention, and Policy, 14*(3), 18.

Williamson, D. F., Madans, J., Anda, R. F., Kleinman, J. C., Giovino, G. A., & Byers, T. (1991). Smoking cessation and severity of weight gain in a national cohort. *New England Journal of Medicine, 324*(11), 739–745.

Wilmore, J. H., Stanforth, P. R., Hudspeth, L. A., Gagnon, J., Daw, E. W., Leon, A. S., et al. (1998). Alterations in resting metabolic rate as a consequence of 20 wk of endurance training: The HERITAGE Family Study. *American Journal of Clinical Nutrition, 68*(1), 66–71.

Wolever, T. M., Jenkins, D. J., Jenkins, A. L., & Josse, R. G. (1991). The glycemic index: Methodology and clinical implications. *American Journal of Clinical Nutrition, 54*(5), 846–854.

Wonderlich, S. A., Rosenfeldt, S., Crosby, R. D., Mitchell, J. E., Engel, S. G., Smyth, J., et al. (2007). The effects of childhood trauma on daily mood lability and comorbid psychopathology in bulimia nervosa. *Journal of Traumatic Stress, 20*(1), 77–87.

World Center for EFT: Emotional Freedom Techniques (n.d.). Retrieved July 9, 2008, from http://www.emofree.com/pdf-files/eftmanual.pdf

World Health Organization and Food and Agriculture Organization (1998). *Carbohydrates in human nutrition: Report of a Joint FAO/WHO Report.* FAO Food and Nutrition Paper 66: Rome.

Wuthrich, B. (2005). Unproven techniques in allergy diagnosis. *Journal of Investigational Allergology and Clinical Immunology, 15*(2), 86–90.

Yapko, M. D. (2003). *Trancework* (3rd ed.). New York: Brunner-Routledge.

Zhao, Y. T., Chen, Q., Sun, Y. X., Li, X. B., Zhang, P., Xy, Y., et al. (2009). Prevention of sudden cardiac death with omega-3 fatty acids in patients with coronary heart disease: A meta-analysis of randomized controlled trials. *Annals of Medicine, 41*(4), 301–10.

Index